THE
PHYSICAL THERAPIST'S
GUIDE
TO HEALTH CARE

THE
PHYSICAL THERAPIST'S
GUIDE
TO HEALTH CARE

Edited by Kathleen A. Curtis, PhD, PT
California State University, Fresno

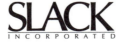

6900 Grove Road • Thorofare, NJ 08086

Publisher: John H. Bond
Editorial Director: Amy E. Drummond
Associate Editor: Jennifer L. Stewart

Curtis, Kathleen
    The physical therapist's guide to health care/edited by Kathleen A. Curtis
        p.   cm.
    Includes bibliographical references and index.
    ISBN 1-55642-378-0 (alk. paper)
    1. Physical therapy--Practice.   2.   Physical therapy--Vocational guid-
ance.
    3. Medical care--United States.   I. Curtis, Kathleen A.
    RM705.P47   1999
    615.8'2'068--dc21   98-46544
                                                                    CIP

Published by: SLACK Incorporated
              6900 Grove Road
              Thorofare, NJ 08086-9447 USA
              Telephone: 609-848-1000
              Fax: 609-853-5991
              World Wide Web: http://www.slackinc.com

Contact SLACK Incorporated for more information about other books in this field or about the availability of our books from distributors outside the United States.

Last digit is print number: 10 9 8 7 6 5 4 3 2 1

TABLE OF CONTENTS

CONTRIBUTING AUTHORS

Kathleen A. Curtis, PhD, PT
Fresno, California

Nichole Hodson-Chennault, MPT
Clovis, California

Wendy Kristy, MPT
Exira, Iowa

Judith M. Reposo, MPT
Fresno, California

Noelle Righter-Freer, MPT
Scotts Valley, California

Julie Roberson, MPT
Fresno, California

Jenna Sawdon, MPT
Fresno, California

Tod Steffenilla, MPT
Monterey, California

Dana Stypula, MPT
Fresno, California

Sonya Yokes, MPT
Carson City, Nevada

ACKNOWLEDGMENTS

The contributors acknowledge Darlene Stewart, MS, PT, Professor Emeritus and former Chairperson, Department of Physical Therapy, California State University, Fresno, for her inspiration, leadership, and landmark work, which validated the role of the academic curriculum in preparing physical therapists for real-world clinical practice. Her book, *Documenting Functional Outcomes in Physical Therapy*, served as the impetus for writing this book and demonstrated the application of new ways of thinking to solve emerging issues and challenges in the physical therapy field.

We also acknowledge Vivian Vidoli, PhD, Dean of the Division of Graduate Studies, California State University, Fresno; Benjamin Cuellar, PhD, Dean of the School of Health and Human Services; and Alexander Gonzalez, PhD, former Provost, California State University, Fresno, for their support of the time required to research, write, and edit this book. This work was funded in part by the 1996-1997 Graduate Student Stipend Program, administered by the Graduate Division, California State University, Fresno, and the 1996-1997 Innovation and Creativity Fund, School of Health and Human Services, California State University, Fresno.

—*Kathleen A. Curtis, PhD, PT*

PREFACE

Recent changes in the health care delivery system have affected practice parameters for all health care providers. Prospective payment systems continue to change mechanisms for health care reimbursement and provide strong incentives for reduced services. Widespread development of health maintenance organizations and preferred provider organizations have forced providers to organize professional networks and provider associations to stay in business. Increasing numbers of our population are underinsured and uninsured, reducing access to needed health care services. Large corporate entities have acquired many smaller hospitals and practices, reducing competition.

This, of course, has had a tremendous impact on the physical therapy profession. Physical therapists have shifted in large numbers from inpatient hospital care to sub-acute, home health, and outpatient settings. Third-party payers have cut back on allowable reimbursement for physical therapy services, and institutions have reduced physical therapy staff positions, leaving fewer professional personnel to manage increasingly larger caseloads.

Clinicians in today's health care environment must not only make sound clinical decisions, they must also develop innovative service delivery mechanisms that respond to the constraints of this changing environment. To effectively do this, they need to have a working knowledge of the structure, policies, constraints, trends and likely future of the health care delivery system. They must have the skills to effectively manage time, their caseloads and multiple support personnel, as well as meet on-going demands for effective documentation, utilization review, quality assurance, and outcomes management. And most importantly, they must be able to envision additional ways to offer and deliver physical therapy services, developing new programs to meet our growing needs for prevention and health promotion.

This book is a practical, strategy-based approach to practice in today's health care environment, specifically written for the physical therapist and physical therapist assistant.

Chapter 1 begins with a discussion of the evolving role of the physical therapist. Chapters 2 and 3 provide an introduction to mechanisms of health care financing, reimbursement, and cost containment. Chapters 4, 5, 6, and 7 focus on physical therapy access issues and trends in three common physical therapy practice settings, including acute, sub-acute and home health care settings. Chapters 8 through 14 provide an in-depth look at professional practice issues, including time management, caseload management and delegation, patient care documentation, measuring outcomes, utilization review, quality assurance, and increasing opportunities for physical therapy in the area of prevention and health promotion.

Although the "rules" may frequently change, physical therapists who can understand the system and see creative avenues to provide patient care services will thrive in the new and changing health care environment. I welcome your insights on how we can effectively meet these challenges.

—Kathleen A. Curtis, PhD, PT

Managing Change

Kathleen A. Curtis, PhD, PT

SPARE CHANGE?

Plenty of it. More than enough to go around in today's health care environment.

In the past decade, there have been widespread changes in the health care delivery system in the United States. National health care reform remains an unresolved issue, as costs continue to rise and payers cut back on reimbursement for services provided. This has significant implications for professional education to prepare clinicians to enter the rapidly changing health care environment.

Physical therapy, as a profession, has been affected in a number of ways that have influenced physical therapists' roles and practice parameters.

Length of Hospital Stay and Shift to Other Levels of Care

We have observed a markedly decreased length of stay of inpatients in hospitals and rehabilitation facilities. Due to decreased lengths of inpatient hospital stays, more services are being delivered in the sub-acute, outpatient, and home health settings.[1-4]

Shortage of Professional Resources

Historically, we have experienced widespread staffing shortages in the face of the rapidly expanding role of physical therapists and the growing elderly population.[5-9] In addition, with recent cost-containment initiatives, physical therapist positions have been cut or restructured, resulting in higher case-loads and increased daily patient volume for remaining staff.

Cost-Containment Strategies

Health care organizations have instituted numerous cost-containment strategies, including training lesser skilled personnel for physical therapy-related functions. Providers now experience strict utilization review with increased accountability to third-party payers and practice in health care environments that are largely funded by prospective payment systems, such as capitation and diagnosis-related group (DRG) reimbursement.[1,2,5,10-17]

Cost-effective and Efficient Outcomes

There is an ever-increasing emphasis on documentation of functional outcomes of physical therapy treatment, especially in relation to costs.[10,18-25] Therapists who have data to support efficient and cost-effective patient management will have an advantage in competing for limited resources.

Shift to Prevention and Wellness

With increasing importance of interventions that promote wellness and prevention of disease and disability, the physical therapist must be concerned not only with providing evaluation and treatment, but also preventing illness and disability. Patient education is, therefore, a critical activity.[4,6,15,16]

Integrated Service Delivery

Integrated service delivery involves interdisciplinary team interaction, collaboration, and coordination between providers to provide professional services to clients and patients with multiple needs. Interdisciplinary case management has been associated with patients reaching higher levels of function in shorter lengths of time.[26] With the increasing complexity of the social service and health care systems, physical therapists cannot meet their patients' needs optimally without working closely with other health care professionals.

Role Changes for the Physical Therapist

The above changes have required a shift in the role of the physical therapist from hands-on treatment to evaluation and assessment, case management, consultation and delegation of treatment responsibilities to others, patient education, documentation, collaboration, and program development.[5-9,21,26,28,29,31]

Understandably, such changes require constant adjustment by the practicing clinician to stay abreast of the health care delivery trends to re-design the related role-specific changes in job responsibilities. Clinicians, educators, and researchers must promote physical therapy and explore alternative methods to meet patient care needs in the changing health care environment.

PRO-ACTIVITY

The purpose of this book is to provide the physical therapist with an orientation to those changes and to empower physical therapists with sufficient knowledge and strategies so that they are able to be pro-active in the current health care environment of the United States.

According to Mel Cohen, PhD, MBA, Financial Manager for Post-acute and Rehabilitation Services, Cedars-Sinai Medical Center, Los Angeles:

Change is easier to accept when it is self-initiated. Those who will be the most successful in a changing environment will greet the need for change with optimism and direct their efforts toward maximizing the gain and minimizing the pain...

As soon as you see change coming, begin work on your foundation. If you need more education or training, go get it. First, to survive and then to thrive, we must accept the inevitability of change. Anticipate the onset of change and take a pro-active stance. Find out what is precipitating the change, clarify your employer's expectations for the outcomes of change, and determine how to implement the change to your advantage.

If you can continue to be an ethical provider of quality care, take whatever steps are required to succeed in the new health care environment. If you choose not to remain, examine your alternatives and initiate the change that will make you a victor rather than a victim. Adjust, adapt, or be gone![27]

WHO'S IN CONTROL OF HEALTH CARE?

Good question! In the past, it was health professionals. Now, many health professionals feel that managed care organizations are determining the type and amount of care that they can provide to consumers.

Cost containment by reducing services? Reducing access to providers? Reducing payment for allowable services? Yes to all of the above.

In some states, providers have contracted with companies who have imposed "gag rules," a clause that prohibits a primary care physician not only from providing secondary referrals and testing, but from even telling the patient that such services exist and might be helpful. Recent ballot proposals in California's 1996 elections saw several proposals directed at limiting the legality of such an arrangement.

Consumers may be losing out as managed care companies profit. The current pendulum swing toward cost containment may soon swing back to a more balanced position. In any case, change is likely, and physical therapists must prepare themselves for a variety of roles—beyond that of providing direct "hands-on" patient care.

CREATING NEW ROLES: SERVICE DELIVERY IN THE MANAGED CARE ENVIRONMENT

Physical therapists who are practicing in today's health care environment must be *present-oriented* and conscious that not only must they live with present-day rules and constraints on practice, but that the rules may change tomorrow, the next day, and even again on the day after that.

Physical Therapist as Evaluator

In an environment with reduced resources, screening and triage become important skills for physical therapists. Screening skills are prioritized evaluative skills. Learning to work smarter, not harder, is the key to performing triage evaluation. The therapist must ask and answer the following questions:

- Which patients need to be seen on a one-on-one basis, and whose needs can be met in a group environment?
- Which patients need daily or twice daily treatment, as opposed to once, twice, or three times weekly, and at what level of care?
- Which patients are changing so rapidly or are so unstable that a professional must constantly reassess the patient responses to treatment before going further?
- What services can be provided by support personnel?
- Which patients have needs that are urgent and should begin services immediately, and which patients can wait?

Physical Therapist as Case Manager

Making these types of decisions requires that physical therapists are aware of the nature of the patient's needs as well as the types of treatment environments (acute, sub-acute, rehabilitation, home health, outpatient) and the skills and capabilities of personnel available to meet those needs.

Responsible case management requires advanced skills in patient advocacy, patient education, and interprofessional communication.

Therapists who are good case managers focus immediately on a discharge plan and what the patient needs to be successful at the next level of care, whether that will be in an institution, outpatient clinic, or in the home. This type of involvement may limit the amount of traditional "hands-on" services that physical therapists can provide.

Strong delegation skills, communication skills, and an organized follow-up system become essential for the physical therapist, as the patient may easily "slip through the cracks" without attention to his or her needs. Only educated health care consumers, who are aware of their needs and how to access adequate care in the medical system, are able to survive in this environment without assistance to navigate. Many patients require strong advocates to empower them, to educate them, and to assist them in accessing the services, equipment, and referrals they need to adequately address their health problems.

Physical Therapist as Consultant

Consultation involves giving your opinion. Physical therapists have been giving their opinions for years, in documenting patient goals and rehabilitation potential, treatment plans, and assessments of patients' progress.

Many physical therapists possess expert knowledge in the field of movement science and pathokinesiology, in rehabilitation, and assistive technology. Some therapists have further specialized in specific clinical domains, sports, industry, long-term care, or with specific patient populations. Others have become experts in health care administration and management.

The consultative role validates one's professional expertise and educates others. It provides understanding of the interrelationships of pathology and functional loss, of impairment and projected outcomes. It relates known research findings to clinical problems. It provides higher level thought processes in the face of a strong movement to reduce service delivery to a series of "cookbook" approaches, critical pathways, and protocols.

Consultation is a critical role for physical therapists to embrace, now and for the future.

Physical Therapist as Educator

Rehabilitation is based on an educational model. Patients and often their care givers *learn* what they need to do to become independent, prevent further disability, maximize their function, reduce pain and stress, and return to work. This learning may occur in the cognitive (thought processes), affective (beliefs, values, and attitudes), and/or psychomotor (movement and skills) domains.

Who better than the physical therapist to provide this education to patients, their families, care givers, supportive personnel, referral sources, and third-party payers? When asked, physical therapists readily acknowledge that education is an important part of what they do.

Many physical therapists, however, fail to validate this role through documentation, out of fear that this is not a "reimbursable" service when in actuality it may make the difference between reoccurrence of disability and continued independence for a patient. In addition, education saves money—for consumers, for their employers, and for third- party payers.

As a profession, physical therapists must become effective educators, understanding health behavior and the factors that tend to motivate and drive human behavior in the health domain. We must avail ourselves of available educational technology, appropriate printed materials, and information systems to have the maximum impact on the patients whom we serve.

Education is the key to prevention and wellness. In a world where more than one-third of our citizens will suffer from disease or disability that can be prevented by diet and exercise, this becomes a critical role for physical therapists to take.

Physical Therapist as Data Analyzer and Outcome Reporter

Documentation. Paperwork. Not a popular subject. This time-consuming function is, however, the key to so much we don't know.

We can learn so much by putting "smart systems" in place to examine our outcomes and the factors that seem to influence them. Paperwork becomes much less of a chore when we have in mind a potential use for the information. We can create systems that serve the needs of patients and third-party payers as well as increasing the knowledge base of our profession by collecting and analyzing outcomes data.

Physical therapists must participate in the development of systems that collect useful, meaningful data on patient function, costs of treatment, types of services provided, and outcomes of treatment. Documentation of this type is the key to providing evidence of the value of our services.

Physical Therapist as Program Developer

With managed health care systems, fewer services may be covered in traditional ways. This requires physical therapists to be creative in providing information and services in nontraditional ways.

Prevention and wellness is one area in which therapists can offer a variety of services, from exercise interventions and sports injury management to workplace productivity, safety, and ergonomic evaluations.

Innovation in service delivery requires physical therapists to be aware of trends and needs of a patient population and be willing to meet these needs in a creative and pro-active manner.

Physical Therapist as Collaborator

With the increasing complexity of our educational, social service, and health care systems, it is not possible for physical therapists to provide for the multiple needs of their patients or clients. Outcomes improve and care is provided more efficiently when professionals from many disciplines collaborate to provide patient- or client-centered services. Further, clients, parents, family members, and care givers need to be included in the collaborative process to explore the optimal solution for each individual client.[28]

Interprofessional collaboration involves working together to reach a common goal in a supportive and mutually beneficial relationship with other team members. Team interactions are characterized by voluntary involvement, parity, and shared decision-making power among team members.[28] Many academic programs are introducing opportunities for students to gain skills in teamwork and interprofessional collaboration.[29-31]

Physical therapists are valuable members of the health care team. Knowledge of organizational and group dynamics, and skills in leadership and communication are at the heart of good teamwork.[28] Your value as an employee and colleague is enhanced by your ability to collaborate.

ABCs OF SUCCESS IN TRANSITION

Act pro-actively, rather than react. Take advantage of opportunities to advance your skills, take on new responsibilities, and try out new ideas. Create systems and organizational structures that will work for the present and future. Set goals and plan to reach them.

Be aware of the big picture. It's easy to get bogged down in details, "being busy," and the hassles and inconveniences of one's daily work. Collect data that help you to analyze the impact of change and innovative approaches and programs. Be brave, be bold.

Change. Be a change agent. Help others to see things differently. Be willing to lead the change process. Be flexible, but also keep in mind what you cannot compromise. Be aware of the legal and ethical implications of change. Educate others. Develop your skills in time management and caseload management. Collaborate with others (including the patient, family, and caregivers) in providing patient services. Challenge yourself with new opportunities to assume new roles in the changing health care environment.

REFERENCES

1. Arthur P. Acute orthopedic services. *PT-Magazine of Physical Therapy.* 1994; 2(6):35-47.
2. Brumfield J. Patient-focused care. *PT-Magazine of Physical Therapy.* 1994; 2(9):76-85, 89.
3. Daus C. Bringing geriatric rehab into the home. *Rehab Management.* 1996; 9(1):53-59.
4. Woods E. Making TRACCS toward a healthier community. *PT-Magazine of Physical Therapy.* 1995; 3(6):40-52.
5. Burcham MR. Managing change. *Rehab Management.* 1994; 7(1):105-106.
6. Coile RC. Forecasting the future. Part One. *Rehab Management.* December/January, 1994; 7(1): 53-56.
7. Daus C. Poised for growth. *Rehab Management.* April/May, 1994; 7(3): 47-49.
8. Forer S. Changing management structures. *Rehab Management.* June/July, 1994; 7(4): 33-38.
9. Selker L. Human resources in physical therapy: Opportunities for service in a rapidly changing health system. *Phys Ther.* 1995;75:31-37.
10. Banja JD. Ethics, outcomes and reimbursement. *Rehab Management.* 1994; 7(1):61-65,136.
11. Clifton DW. A shift toward utilization management. *PT-Magazine of Physical Therapy.* 1995;3(6):32-35.
12. Clifton DW, Tecklin JS. Under the watchful eye. *Rehab Management.* 1995; 8(1):43-47.
13. Foto M, Swanson G. Utilization review and managed care. *Rehab Management.* 1993; 6(5):123-124.
14. Hunter SJ, Olsen B, Stewart L. TQM in PT. *PT-Magazine of Physical Therapy.* 1993; 1(7):54-58,85.
15. Monahan B. Managing under managed care phase II. *PT-Magazine of Physical Therapy.* 1995;3(7):38-47.
16. Monahan B. Managing under managed care. *PT-Magazine of Physical Therapy.* 1993; 1(7):34-40.
17. Woods EN. Restructuring of America's hospitals: What does it mean for physical therapy. *PT-Magazine of Physical Therapy.* 1994; 2(6):34-41.
18. Benton S. Uniform data system for medical rehabilitation. *Rehab Management.* 1994; 7(6):13.
19. Daus C. Quantifying outcomes through clinical research. *Rehab Management.* 1994; 7(4):143-146.

20. Forer S. Outcomes evaluation in sub-acute care. *Rehab Management.* 1995;8(4):1138-1140,1164.
21. Jette AM. Outcomes research: Shifting the dominant research paradigm in physical therapy. *Phys Ther.* 1995;7(75):965-970.
22. Moore RW, Salcido R. Rehabilitation outcomes in subacute care. *Rehab Management.* Dec/Jan, 1996; 9(1):97-111.
23. Reynolds JP. What is the outcomes movement? What does it mean to PTs. *PT-Magazine of Physical Therapy.* 1995; 3(7):49-52, 67-68.
24. Wilkerson D. Developing outcomes management tools. *Rehab Management.* 1995; 8(1):114-177,129.
25. Wilkerson D. Implementing outcomes. *Rehab Management.* 1995; 8(6):97-99,116.
26. Erickson B, Perkins M. Interdisciplinary team approach in the rehabilitation of hip and knee arthroplasties. *Am J Occup Ther.* 1994; 48(5):429-441.
27. Cohen M. Got any spare change. *Advance for Physical Therapists (editorial).* 1996; 3: 62.
28. O'Connor B. Challenges of interagency collaboration: Serving a young child with severe disabilities. In: McEwen IR, ed. *Occupational and Physical Therapy in Educational Environments.* New York: Haworth Press, Inc., 1995.
29. Hilton RW, Morris DJ, Wright AM. Learning to work in the health care team. *Journal of Interprofessional Care.* 1995;9(3):267-274.
30. Richardson J, Edwards M. An undergraduate clinical skills laboratory developing interprofessional skills in physical and occupational therapy. *Gerontology and Geriatrics Education.* 1997; 17(4):33-43.
31. MacKinnen JL, MacRae N. Fostering geriatric interdisciplinary collaboration through academic education. *Physical and Occupational Therapy in Geriatrics.* 1996; 14(3):41-49.

TEST YOUR SKILLS

What are the implications for physical therapists, for patients, and for third-party payers of each of the following trends mentioned in Chapter 1?

Trend	For PTs	For Patients	For Third-Party Payers
Length of hospital stay and shift to other levels of care			
Shortage of professional resources			
Cost containment strategies			
Cost-effective and efficient outcomes			
Shift to prevention and wellness			
Integrated services delivery			
Role changes for the physical therapist			

CHECK YOUR RESPONSES

Trend	For PTs	For Patients	For Third-Party Payers
Length of hospital stay and shift to other levels of care	Evaluation, goal-setting, and discharge decision must be made quickly. Sound case management may require delegation of routine care to multi-skilled personnel. Priority is on preparing the patient for the next level of care.	Potential for discontinuity of care upon discharge. Patient and family need to be included in goal-setting and the discharge planning process. Need education on appropriate physical therapy services and equipment to meet goals.	Lower costs associated with home health care and skilled nursing facility care. Needs educating about the patient's condition and needs for physical therapy services at all levels of care.
Shortage of professional resources	Strong patient advocacy required in documenting why professional physical therapist skills are required for patient's needs. Requires solid footing in ethical and legal requirements for delegation of patient care responsibilities to support personnel.	Possible lack of continuity of care for the patient. Less time with therapist; more time with support personnel. More time in classes or group treatment settings. Needs more education.	Costs are lower when support personnel provide services. Needs education to understand how a professional's judgment and skills differ from routine services provided by multi-skilled support personnel.
Cost containment strategies	External authorization to provide services may limit frequency and duration of services provided and requires strong patient advocacy skills. Documentation must be up to date and accurately reflect the patient's need for physical therapy services. Therapists must be pro-active and creative in suggesting more cost-efficient ways to provide PT services.	Unable to access needed services. Early discharge from health care facilities may shift burden of care onto family members or require hospitalization in long-term care and skilled nursing facilities.	Frequently institutes measures (utilization review or utilization management) to authorize payment (either retrospectively or prospectively) for physical therapy services. Needs education to understand how a professional's judgment and skills differ from routine services provided by multi-skilled support personnel.
Cost-effective and efficient outcomes	Physical therapists must collect data that shows the time required and associated costs to achieve functional outcomes. Value and efficiency are gaining in importance in competing for limited resources.	Patients perceive greater value in returning to work and activities faster and at less out-of-pocket costs.	Want to work with providers who provide appropriate, time-efficient, and cost-effective services.

Trend	For PTs	For Patients	For Third-Party Payers
Shift to prevention and wellness	Physical therapists need to fully develop their role in health promotion and screening, including such areas as prevention of injuries, falls, and repetitive strain in the home and workplace, child development, fitness, and women's health issues.	Patients will benefit by not needing services after an injury that has been prevented. Early intervention is often less costly and involved and provides for easier lifestyle modification. Consumers save money on costs of insurance, medication, and diagnostic and treatment services.	Will potentially save money by the implementation of widespread disease and injury prevention programs.
Integrated services delivery	Requires a commitment to interprofessional teamwork, communication, and shared decision making.	Provides a more efficient path to desired goals. Coordinates care giver approaches to simplify intervention for patient and family.	May provide "bundling" of services, which shifts risk to provider groups. Patients reach goals faster, which reduces costs of institutionalization.
Role changes for the physical therapist	Requires advanced and continuing education to stay abreast of changes in health care. Therapists must develop efficient screening and evaluative skills. Case management, consultation, collaboration, delegation, patient education, and program development skills will become priorities in recruiting, retaining, and promoting physical therapists.	Patients must be introduced to members of the health care team and understand what role the physical therapist plays in providing and supervising patient care services. The patient may work less intensively (on an ongoing basis) with the physical therapist and more in group settings or with supportive personnel.	Need education to understand physical therapist educational background, sound rationale and data for treatment recommendations, practice guidelines, program development, and patient education programs. If physical therapists do not take proactive roles in fostering this educational process, the third-party payers will make their own decisions.

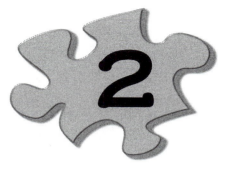

BASICS OF HEALTH CARE FINANCING AND REIMBURSEMENT

Wendy Kristy, MPT

Two important concepts in health care are *financing* and *reimbursement*. The aim of this chapter is to familiarize the reader with these concepts and how they influence the delivery of physical therapy services.

Health care *financing* is the flow of dollars from individual enrollees, employers, or the government to a health plan. In contrast, *reimbursement* is considered the flow of dollars from a health plan to a provider (Figure 2.1).[1]

THE FOUR BASIC TYPES OF HEALTH CARE FINANCING

There are four basic ways that health care is paid for in the United States: *out-of-pocket payments*, *individual private insurance*, *employment-based private insurance*, and *government financing*.

Figure 2.2 illustrates the percentage of the US population enrolled in various health care plans. In 1995, only 9% of the US population was covered by individual private health insurance. Most of the population has relied on other forms of health insurance, such as employment-based private insurance (61%) and government-subsidized insurance (25%). An additional 15% were uninsured.[2]

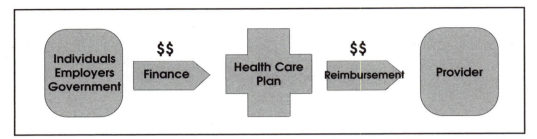

FIGURE 2.1 *Financing and reimbursing of health care. Adapted with permission from Bodenheimer TS, Grumbach K.* Understanding health policy: a clinical approach. *Norwalk, Conn: Appleton & Lange; 1995.*

Out-of-Pocket Payments

Out-of-pocket financing of health care is similar to buying groceries at the grocery store. This was the original way that health care was financed. Forty or 50 years ago, many physicians practiced house calls, visiting sick patients in their homes. Patients and families paid physicians out of the pocket for their services. *Out-of-pocket* payment is reimbursement by the means of the patient or patient's family and is simply a direct purchase by the consumer for the services or goods rendered. This out-of-pocket payment is usually based on a *fee-for-service* (FFS) or a reduced fee-for-service arrangement.

Today, consumers purchase what they need and want with the out-of-pocket payment method. Consider some of the items we often purchase (CD players, VCRs, computers). We spend our money on such luxury items without a second thought except, perhaps, to be sure we are getting the best our money can buy. This is not, however, the way that health care is purchased in the United States.

Unlike luxury items, Americans as a whole consider health care to be a basic human right[1,3] and, therefore, are not willing to pay out-of-pocket for it. The general attitude is that health care is a right for all people, and all who need it (including the under-employed, sick, and elderly) must receive it whether or not they have the resources to pay for it. This attitude makes paying for health care a challenge, particularly because the need for health care is unpredictable and can be extremely costly.

Health care is now available to more people; both access and technology have been improved tremendously over the past three decades. However, with these improvements, costs have increased markedly, making pure out-of-pocket payments an impossible method for financing health care for most Americans.[1] As a result, other methods of financing have emerged to make medical care more affordable and accessible to more people.

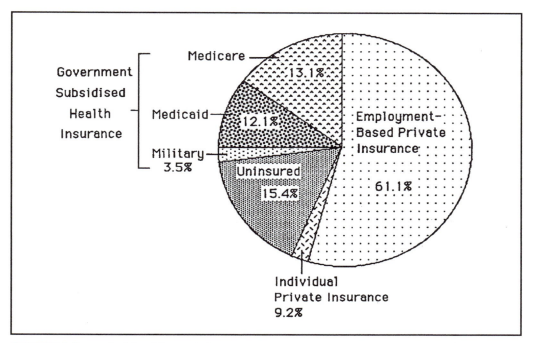

FIGURE 2.2 *Percent of the US population covered by various health care plans in 1995. Note: The estimates by type of coverage are not mutually exclusive; in other words, individuals can be covered by more than one type of health insurance during the year. Source: US Bureau of the Census, March 1996 Current Population Survey.*

Individual Private Insurance

Health care purchased by an individual is called *individual private insurance*. Here a third party is added, dividing payments into two transactions: financing and reimbursement (see Figure 2.1).

Individual private insurance is financed by the subscriber who agrees to pay an out-of-pocket monthly premium to a health insurance company in exchange for a defined set of medical services. To receive insurance benefits, the subscriber must seek medical services from only those providers who are covered under the plan that they have purchased. The subscriber must also pay for any medical charges, such as deductibles, copayments, and services not covered by the plan.

Additional medical charges

- **Deductible:** a designated amount of medical charges that must be paid by the subscriber to the provider before the insurance company will pay for remaining charges.

- **Copayment:** a designated amount of money that the subscriber pays directly to the provider at each visit.
- **Uncovered services:** those services that are not paid for by the insurance company.

Many individual private insurance plans include an indemnity clause that allows the subscriber to see a provider outside of the insurance plan. This allows the enrollee to seek medical care from a provider who is not included in the plan, but it typically requires a higher out-of-pocket expense to the enrollee. Consider the following example of how indemnity insurance may be used:

Leigh Whitehall pays $200 per month for her health insurance. She was given a list of providers, including physical therapists, for which the insurance company covers 80% of all costs. Over the course of time, she developed tendonitis in the elbow and obtained a physician referral for physical therapy. She shared this information with a friend, who told her of a similar problem she had experienced just 2 years earlier, and how she was treated by a "PT who really knows his stuff." Leigh decided she wanted to be treated by this physical therapist but found he was not on her list of approved providers. Leigh considered that, instead of paying only 20% of the charges, she would have to pay 50%, because the therapist she wanted to be treated by was not an approved provider. She decided to see the recommended therapist and was charged $60 for her first visit.

Employment-Based Private Insurance

Initial forms of private insurance appeared just prior to (and during) the Great Depression, when hospitals were unable to attract customers. Hospital costs were rising because of advances in technology and effectiveness of care, which made out-of-pocket payments unrealistic for most people. In addition, the Depression made it even more difficult for patients to pay for their health care and, subsequently, the number of occupants in private hospitals decreased.

To increase utilization, hospitals made themselves more accessible by creating prepayment plans for certain groups of people that allowed a predetermined amount of hospital coverage; hence, private health insurance was born. At first, specific hospitals required that care be provided at their facilities only. However, by the late 1930s, Blue Cross (covering hospital expenses) and Blue Shield (covering physician services) offered a choice of providers to consumers.

During World War II, there arose a shortage of workers, as many were sent off to fight in the war. In an effort to attract workers, rival companies began a "wage war," in which employers competed with each other for workers. As a result, the government imposed a wage freeze, which prevented employers from increasing wages to attract workers. At this time, employers began to sponsor health insurance for their employees as part of a fringe benefit package; hence, employer-sponsored health insurance came to be.

Employment-based health insurance became very popular and attracted many new insurance plans to compete with Blue Cross and Blue Shield. It was during this era that competition among insurance plans took on new approaches. One approach, called *experience rating*, involved the classification of groups of workers (prospective subscribers) into various utilization levels. For example, accountants typically used fewer health care services than did coal miners. By determining the level of utilization of different groups, insurance premiums were determined.[1] Consider the following scenario:

Healthland Insurance Company insures three groups of people using experience rating: young and healthy accountants, older and healthy teachers, and older coal miners with a high rate of chronic black lung disease. Healthland charges premiums to subscribers according to the experience of the group to which they belong. According to experience rating, the accountants had the lowest utilization rate of medical services and, therefore, were charged a premium of $100. The older teachers were charged $300 for their premiums because, according to experience rating, older groups tend to use medical services more. The older coal miners were charged $500 for their premium because not only were they older, but their job was associated with a higher rate of health care utilization due to chronic black lung disease. The average premium income for Healthland was $300 per member per month.

Experience rating may seem more fair to groups who are healthy and who don't feel they should be paying for someone else's health care. However, experience rating decreases the availability of health care to higher risk groups (those who are under-employed, poor, and chronically ill) by discriminating against them through higher premium charges.

Another approach, *community rating*, bases health care on human need instead of anticipated use. For example, premiums would be even for all groups, but excess money from premiums of healthy groups would go toward subsidizing the "sicker" groups who were unable to fully cover their costs.[1]

Initially, private health insurance companies typically used experience ratings to attract low-risk groups, whereas Blue Cross and Blue Shield used community ratings to distribute health care according to need among groups.

> *WeCare Health Insurance Company insures a similar mix of subscriber groups as does Healthland and requires $300 per month to cover member expenses and administration. Instead of experience rating, WeCare uses community rating to determine premiums. The premium for each of the three groups (young and healthy accountants, older and healthy restaurant managers, older factory workers with a high rate of chronic back problems) is the same, regardless of the anticipated utilization of medical services.*

Eventually, however, private insurance companies won out because their plans were affordable to more people, forcing Blue Cross and Blue Shield to use experience rating in order to maintain their place in the health care market. Subsequently, groups of people who used more health care (ie, the elderly and chronically ill) became less able to pay for their medical needs. From the perspective of those who use more health care services, the practice of experience rating is discriminatory and makes access to health care more difficult.

Figure 2.1 also illustrates how employment-based private health insurance is financed. In 1995, 61% of the US population financed its health care through employment-based private insurance. With this form of health insurance, employers usually pay all or part of the premium that purchases health insurance for their employees.[1] It has been shown, however, that full coverage, in which the employer pays everything for employee health care, leads to higher utilization of services and thus higher costs.[1,4] Employers, therefore, now typically pay a specified percentage (ie, 80%) of the lowest cost plan offered while the employee is responsible for the remaining costs.

Government-Financed Health Care

Although private insurance (individual and employment-based) was abundant by the late 1950s, it did not insure all who needed health care. Specifically, the poor and elderly had little resources to access health care, especially with experience-rated insurance premiums for these groups. For this reason, the development of Medicare and Medicaid programs began, and, in 1965, the Social Security Act was passed.

As shown in Figure 2.3, a new feature was introduced into health care financing: the taxpayer. The government began to subsidize health care plans, which are known as the Medicare and Medicaid programs. These public plans have helped to increase access to health care immensely. For example, during the late 1950s, less than 15% of the elderly population had any health insurance. The enactment of the Medicare and Medicaid programs helped to provide health insurance to nearly 85% of all Americans by 1966.[5]

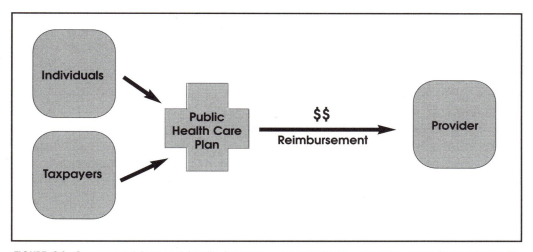

FIGURE 2.3 *Government-financed health insurance. Adapted with permission from Bodenheimer TS, Grumbach K.* Understanding health policy: a clinical approach. *Norwalk, Conn: Appleton & Lange; 1995.*

To be eligible for Medicare, an individual must be a citizen or permanent resident of the United States who has worked and contributed to Social Security for at least 10 years and is at least 65 years of age. Citizens younger than 65 are entitled to Medicare if they have been receiving Social Security benefits for 24 months or have end-stage renal disease. A person can also be eligible if his or her spouse has met the employment requirement.[6]

Traditionally, Medicare consisted of two plans, Part A and Part B. Medicare Part A ("inpatient" or "hospital insurance") is financed largely through Social Security taxes from employers and employees, whereas Medicare Part B ("outpatient" or "physician services") is financed through federal taxes and monthly premiums from the subscribers.[1] Medicare Part A pays for the cost of a medically necessary stay in an inpatient hospital, skilled nursing facility, or hospice, and it pays for home health care. Medicare Part B pays for the cost of medically necessary physicians' services and other medical services and supplies, such as physical therapy, x-rays, immunizations, ambulance transportation, and durable medical equipment (DME).[6]

More recently, the Balanced Budget Act of 1997 was passed, and Medicare Part C was added to give individuals entitled to Medicare Part A and enrolled under Part B the ability to elect to receive benefits through the existing Medicare Part B program or a Medicare + Choice plan. The Medicare + Choice options include:

- coordinated care plans (including health maintenance organizations [HMOs], preferred provider organizations [PPOs], and similar arrangements)
- plans offered by provider-sponsored organizations (PSOs)

- a combination of a medical savings account (MSA) plan and contributions to a Medicare + Choice MSA
- private fee-for-service (FFS) plans[7,8]

Medicaid (MediCal in California) is a state-administered program that provides medical assistance to the poor and is financed through both state and federal taxes.[1] Ironically, the taxpayers who contribute to this program usually exceed income requirements for eligibility. In general, healthy taxpayers pay more into the Medicare/Medicaid system than they use, while the unemployed, elderly, and disabled pay less (or nothing) and use it more.

Several factors led to an increase in government-subsidized health care expenditures, including unemployment, high costs of health care, a rapidly growing elderly population, and increased lifespan of those with chronic conditions.[1,9] Medicaid expenditures, in particular, have increased; and with the weakening economy, there was an increase in the number of people who were financially eligible for this government assistance.[2] Even though Medicare and Medicaid improved financial access to health care for the vast majority of elderly needy people, it has also aggravated the problem of rising costs.

HOW HEALTH CARE PROVIDERS ARE REIMBURSED

In this section, basic payment methods, financial risk, how providers are reimbursed, and how reimbursement influences provider behavior in health care will be discussed.

Remember that *reimbursement* is the flow of money from health insurance companies to providers (ie, physicians, hospitals, allied health professionals) (see Figure 2.1). The United States has a complex payment system with a variety of rules dictating how providers are reimbursed.

First, it is important for a provider to know whether the rate of reimbursement is negotiated after the services have been provided (*retrospective payment*) or before the services have been provided (*prospective payment*). Almost all reimbursement prior to the 1980s was done retrospectively. This led to rapidly increasing health costs as provider fees for health care services and use of high-cost technologies escalated. With the onset of *prospective payment systems (PPS)*, payers became increasingly involved in setting limits, rates, and methods by which they would reimburse providers.

Second, the provider should know how provider services are *bundled* or grouped for reimbursement and the *financial risks and incentives* associated with each method of reimbursement. There are four basic reimbursement methods commonly used today. These methods include *fee for service, per visit, per case or episode*, and *capitation*.

Fee For Service (FFS)

With *fee-for-service (FFS) reimbursement*, each fee is directly associated with a service. This method of payment is much like grocery shopping, in that you pay the indicated price for each item you have in your grocery basket. For example, a patient who is referred to a physical therapist and receives electrical stimulation, moist heat, and therapeutic exercise would be charged for these services according to a set fee schedule. The fee schedule is based on what is usual, customary, and reasonable (UCR).

Per Visit

With *per-visit reimbursement*, the provider is reimbursed a specific amount each time a patient is treated. This method is not as closely associated with specific services provided as FFS reimbursement. When providers are paid per visit, they have a stronger incentive to not exceed appropriate levels of care within a single patient visit.[2] Over-treating patients decreases the potential volume of patients who can be treated and, therefore, puts the provider at risk of losing income.

Per Case or Per Episode

Payment per case or per episode simply means that providers are given one payment for each episode or hospital admission, often by the diagnosis for which a patient requires medical intervention. This payment method bundles more services into one payment than both FFS and per-visit methods by being more related to a patient's condition or diagnosis. An example of this method of payment is Medicare diagnosis-related groups (DRGs), in which a predetermined fee is paid to the acute hospital provider for each admission by patient diagnosis. When physical therapy services are typically required (ie, total joint replacements), the hospital provider is given an additional amount to account for these services.

However, diagnosis by itself is often a poor predictor of rehabilitation needs; therefore, this payment method puts providers at greater risk of losing money.[10,11] For example, the least complicated patients will most likely cost less than the per episode reimbursement allowance, thereby creating a margin of profit for the provider. In contrast, the more complicated patients will substantially exceed the reimbursement allowance and create a financial loss for the provider. This gives the provider the incentive to find healthier populations to treat, which often translates to targeting groups with higher socio-economic status and healthy elderly populations.

Capitation

Capitation is essentially unrelated to services provided.[10] With capitation, one payment for each health plan member is paid each month (or year), regardless of the utilization of services by that member. This is also known as a *per-member-per-month* (PMPM) payment system. According to Jim Nugent, "in comparing all payment systems under managed care, capitation puts the provider at the greatest risk" for operating at a financial loss.[10]

Bundling services and shifting risk

Methods of payment are on a continuum that range from being the least bundled (ie, FFS) to the most bundled (ie, capitation). Bundling is the grouping of services relative to a specific fee a provider is paid.[10] Figure 2.4 illustrates the level of bundling with each method of reimbursement.

An unbundled payment is closely linked to the services that are provided, such as FFS. Here, the charges are added up according to what specific services were provided. For example, $15 for moist hot packs, $25 for soft tissue mobilization, and $25 for therapeutic exercise would add up to a $65 charge.

In a bundled payment method, reimbursement is dependent on the number of patient visits or type of diagnosis treated. For example, a bundled payment is similar to paying for the typical all-you-can-eat salad bar. No matter how much salad you eat, the cost is the same because it is prepaid and not connected to how much is eaten. Capitation, salary, and global budgets are examples of bundled payment methods.

Figure 2.4 shows current payment methods ranging from the least to the most bundled.

As payment plans become more bundled, financial risk shifts to the provider. Financial risk refers to the potential to lose money, earn less money, or spend more time without additional payment on reimbursement transactions.[1] Using the salad bar example, the restaurant owner is at risk for losing money when there is a single price for unlimited services. If customers eat a lot of the more expensive items, the owner may lose money.

Figure 2.4 illustrates how fee-for-service transactions put all the risk on the payer and capitation puts all the risk on the provider. Consider the scenario on Page 23.

In this scenario, we see how the provision of physical therapy services is influenced by a capitated reimbursement method. In order to break even, David decides to limit how many services he offers at each patient visit. In all

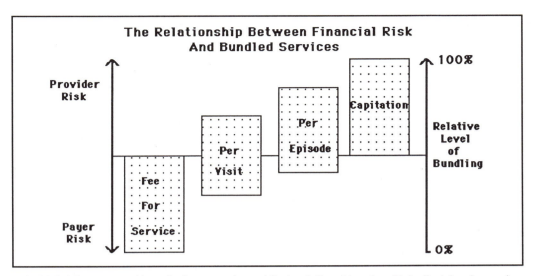

FIGURE 2.4 *Summary of bundled payments and their relative risk value. Note that fee-for-service payments put all financial risk on the payer, while at the same time it remains the least bundled payment method. Capitation places all risk on the provider, while at the same time it is the most bundled method of reimbursement. Salary and global budgets are other methods of bundled payments that put risk on the provider.*

David Sellick is a physical therapist with his own practice. He contracts with an insurance company that reimburses him $50 per patient visit. This amount of reimbursement is just enough to cover his costs for space, utilities, and support staff. David strives to limit his treatments to 30 minutes per patient to make ends meet, but his more complicated patients require more treatment time and services. He realizes that he will not be paid for these additional services and subsequently is forced to take a financial loss.

types of physical therapy settings, however, some patients need more care than others. In David's case, having enough patients who need less care will help balance out those who need more care. It would be prudent of David to be pro-active and find out which treatment protocols are more efficient and effective.

Managed Care Players

In this section, three forms of managed care coverage and how they typically carry out the reimbursement process will be discussed. Three common examples of managed care coverage for health care services are FFS with utilization review, PPOs, and HMOs.

Fee-for-service reimbursement with utilization review

This is the traditional FFS payment system with a twist of third-party payer involvement. Third-party payers (ie, an insurance company or government agency) review patient records after treatment has been rendered and decide whether or not the services provided fall under UCR standards. If services meet UCR criteria, the insurance company will reimburse the provider. If the services do not meet UCR standards, then payment is denied. In short, this managed care plan gives the insurer the right to deny reimbursement.[1]

Preferred provider organization

A *PPO* is an arrangement in which a specific group of providers agree to provide services for their subscribers at a negotiated FFS rate, which is usually less than their normal rate. Although payments under this system are discounted, providers gain referrals and, therefore, can potentially increase revenue by seeing more patients. Providers typically belong to at least one or more PPOs in an effort to maximize their referral base.

Health Maintenance Organization

An HMO is an organization that combines insurers and providers into one entity. Both FFS with utilization review and PPOs use retrospective payments (payments made after services have been provided). In contrast, an HMO is a prepaid group practice. The enrollee pays a fixed fee and in return receives a specific set of health care benefits.[1] With the exception of emergencies, patients who enroll in an HMO are generally required to receive their care within a particular HMO. The provider's reimbursement is usually more bundled (ie, per diem or per day, capitation, or salary) and, therefore, changes the incentive from "treat more, be paid more" to "treat less, be paid the same."

Gatekeeping is a common feature within many HMO plans. While serving as first contact for the patient and then determining the need for specialized services, the primary care physician (gatekeeper) provides continuity and coordination of patient care.

Consider these two types of HMOs:

Independent practice association (IPA) model HMOs are loose networks of private providers and hospitals. An IPA contracts with an HMO and serves as an intermediate level of reimbursement (Figure 2.5). Usually a gatekeeper (or primary physician) is used to direct the care of patients and has control over health care costs by using an efficient referral system.

Group or staff model HMOs bring all providers under one roof. Kaiser

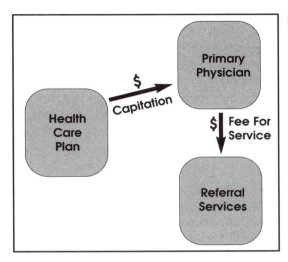

FIGURE 2.5 *Two-tiered capitation structure. The health plan reimburses the primary physician via capitation. The primary physician is then at risk for paying for referral services out of his or her own capitation income. Adapted with permission from Bodenheimer TS, Grumbach K.* Understanding Health Policy: A Clinical Approach. *Norwalk, Conn: Appleton & Lange; 1995.*

Permanente is an example of a staff model HMO. All providers are housed under one roof so that patients can go to the same facility for all care (ie, routine physician visits, emergencies, surgeries, laboratory tests, x-rays, immunizations, and hospital admissions). In the staff model HMO, the providers are employed by the HMO. Here, too, a gatekeeper is used to ensure appropriate patient care.

Many providers will contract with a variety of payer sources, giving any one provider multiple and varying forms of reimbursement. Consider the following scenario:

Sharon Wesley runs her own physical therapy practice in a busy suburb. She contracts with several payers, including Sunrise Health Foundation, Livelong Medical Insurance, and Tri-Valley Health Care. On November 1, 1995, she was scheduled to see three patients who were referred from each one of these insurance companies.

At 9 am, Jack Milton, a patient with low back pain, arrived. He is insured by Sunrise Health Foundation, a local insurance company that reimburses FFS after utilization review. The following services were provided for the given FFS charges: moist heat ($30), electrical stimulation ($60), ultrasound ($45), soft tissue mobilization ($35), therapeutic exercises ($80), and ice massage ($25). The total charges ($305) were billed to Sunrise Health Foundation and awaited review and payment.

At 10 am, Barkley Wallace arrived to be treated for his low back pain. His insurance carrier is Livelong Medical Insurance, a large PPO in the area. Sharon offers the same treatment protocol to Barkley as she did for Jack, but the charges were discounted to honor her contract with the PPO. Livelong Medical Insurance was charged $150.

Continued on Page 26

After lunch, Sharon's 1:30 pm patient, Stephen Garcia, arrived to be treated for low back pain. He is insured by Tri-Valley Health Care, which is an HMO that pays via capitation. Sharon provided a slightly different treatment session for Stephen in order to keep her costs down. Instead of using isokinetic exercises, she taught the patient exercises he can do at home and referred him to her "back school" session the following Wednesday. Instead of providing ice massage, she has an aide place an ice pack on his low back after exercising. As a result, her time with this patient was less "hands-on" and more instructive. Sharon does not bill Tri-Valley Health Care for this session because she already receives a PMPM payment.

Six weeks later, when Sharon reviewed the prior month's financial records, she noted payments she received for the three patients she treated on November 1, 1995.

Patient	Insurance Type	Charge	Payment received
Jack Milton	FFS	$305	$225
Barkley Wallace	PPO	$150	$150
Stephen Garcia	HMO	$200	$1.00

In this scenario, Sharon receives the most payment from the FFS insurance, although it is not the full amount charged. This amount received is reflective of the amount Sunrise Health Foundation decided was the UCR charge. She received the same amount that was charged from the PPO because full reimbursement of discounted services is part of the PPO contract. In contrast, she received only $1 from the HMO, even though the cost to Sharon was $200. It appears that Sharon was not paid for treating her HMO patient. However, this is misleading because Sharon also received $1.00 for each of her other patients covered by the HMO who did not receive physical therapy treatment that month.

Physician Reimbursement

Physicians are reimbursed for their services by third-party payers by *fee for service, per visit, per episode*, and *capitation methods*.

Fee for service

FFS payment has been the traditional source of reimbursement to physicians until the cost-containment era (see Chapter 10). Today, the UCR approach to fee setting has been replaced by payer-determined fee schedules, such as those used in Medicaid, Medicare, and PPOs.

For example, for a typical office visit, Medicaid pays only what is on its fee schedule for that service, even if the actual cost is greater. Medicaid might only pay $16 for an office visit even though the actual charge is $45.

In contrast, the Medicare system has used a *resource-based relative-value fee schedule (RBRVS)*. This system sets fees based on the time, mental effort and judgment, technical skill, physical effort, and stress typically related to the service.[1,8] Similarly, PPOs typically pay physicians with whom they have contracted on a discounted FFS schedule.

With FFS payment, the physician has the incentive to provide more services because more revenue can potentially be generated. This can (and has) become a problem with over-utilization creating increased costs for the payer (see Chapter 12). Prospective payment and bundled payment methods address this issue.

Payment per episode

Under managed care plans, surgeons are typically reimbursed with a bundled payment, as in *payment per episode*. As previously illustrated, this transfers some risk from the payer to the provider. Consider the following scenario:

> *Peter Jones just underwent a total knee replacement for which Dr. Smith was paid $7000. This payment was based on average surgical costs for this procedure and five postoperative follow-up visits. However, after his surgery, Peter developed an infection that required antibiotic management and wound debridement with secondary closure. This extended his care by months and required 30 additional office visits. Dr. Smith was not paid for the additional time and charges that were accrued as a result of Mr. Jones' complication.*

Per-episode reimbursement provides an incentive for surgeons to conduct more surgeries and limit the number of follow-up visits postoperatively. In addition, there is an added incentive to spend very little time with each patient per visit. In this way, they limit costs and maximize profits. In contrast, FFS payment strategies would provide an incentive for a longer duration of follow-up care and more procedures per visit, which would increase revenue by increasing the frequency and volume of services to an individual patient.

Payment per patient

Capitation: two-tiered structure

In the United States, the two-tiered health care structure exists in a small

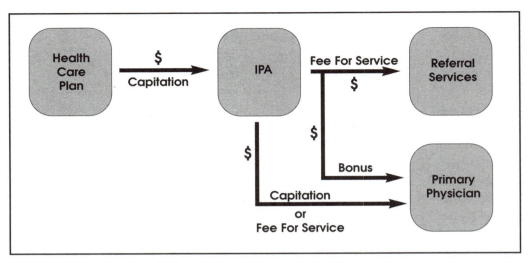

FIGURE 2.6 *Three-tiered capitation structure. When both the IPA and primary physician are reimbursed via capitated payments, the physician may receive a bonus if the IPA realizes a year-end surplus in its budget for referral services. When the IPA reimburses its primary physicians on a fee-for-service basis, a portion of the total predetermined fee is paid (ie, 60%). If money is left over at the end of the year, the physicians receive a portion of the withheld monies as a bonus. Adapted with permission from Bodenheimer TS, Grumbach K.* Understanding Health Policy: A Clinical Approach. *Norwalk, Conn: Appleton & Lange; 1995.*

percentage of all HMOs (approximately 20%). The first tier is the health care plan, and the second tier is the primary physician. The health plan pays the primary care physician directly via a monthly capitated fee. Any referred services are then paid directly by the health plan via an FFS method. Under this system, the more members enrolled with a primary physician, the more money that physician makes, regardless of the volume of patients seen or the number of outside referrals that physician makes (see Figure 2.5).[1,12]

Capitation: three-tiered structure

The remaining HMOs in the United States are generally made up of groups of physicians or small group practices (IPAs). In this arrangement, the first tier (the HMO) reimburses the second tier (the administrative physician group or IPA) via full or partially capitated payments. The third tier (member physicians) is reimbursed either by capitated or FFS payments (the payment method is determined by the IPA). The locus of control, therefore, lies with the physician group, not with the HMOs. Physicians in these groups share the financial risk and will profit from patients enrolled in an HMO only if the cost to the group for use of services is lower than capitated payments.[13] This payment structure is shown in Figure 2.6.

Consider the case in which the IPA pays for referral services via capitated

fees. This spreads the financial risk throughout the organization's participants, thus reducing the risk borne by individual primary physicians. These
physicians often have a built-in incentive to reduce their overall use of specialist services by way of a year-end bonus. The fewer referrals made, the less
money spent, and the more money remains in balance, leaving a larger year-
end bonus for the primary physicians.

In the case in which an FFS payment is made by the IPA for referred services (to a specialist physician), more risk is placed on the IPA because the FFS
charges from the referral services can easily surpass their initial capitated
reimbursement. To minimize their risk, the IPA typically will only reimburse a
portion of the fees charged (eg, 60%) and will withhold the rest (eg, 40%). If
money is left over at the end of the year, the group of specialists (referred services) receive a portion of the withheld money as a bonus. Therefore, even
though the IPA is mostly at risk, all involved physicians share in the risk by
having an incentive to not overspend or over-utilize specialists.

Hospital Reimbursement

Payment per procedure

The *payment per procedure* (equivalent to fee for service) reimbursement
method has been the traditional method of hospital payment for private hospitals. However, this method has not been as prevalent since the "reasonable
cost" system has been implemented. To a large extent, hospitals were allowed
to determine their charges under this system.

Because of cost control issues, private and public payers have begun to
question the "reasonable costs" of hospitals. As a result of financial risk, there
has been a shift from FFS forms of payment to per diem, per episode (DRG),
and capitation payments.

Payment per diem (per day)

In this payment method, the hospital is paid a set amount per day.
Therefore, the number of days a patient is in the hospital puts the payer at
risk, whereas the number of services performed puts the provider at risk.
Consider the scenario on Page 30.

The *per-diem* method of payment bundles the services for 1 day into one
payment. If few or no expensive tests are performed, the hospital could make
a profit. However, if many expensive tests are performed, the hospital's costs
go up, and the hospital could lose money. Therefore, a representative of
Medicaid reviews the use of services (ie, utilization review) in order to reduce
the number days patients stay in the hospital. In fact, HMOs that provide

Michael Morales, a Medicaid patient, is admitted to the hospital with severe chest pain. He has continuous electrocardiogram (EKG) monitoring, blood tests, a chest x-ray, coronary angiography, and an angioplasty with stent placement performed during his stay. The doctors determine he has sustained a small myocardial infarction and put him on beta blockers and a nitroglycerin patch for ongoing management. His condition improves, and he is sent home 3 days later. Medicaid reimburses the hospital $700 per day, or $2100. Based on an FFS payment schedule, the cost of Mr. Morales' stay is $5400.

Hugh Holland, another Medicaid patient who has a history of hypertension, is admitted to the hospital with congestive heart failure. He receives intravenous medications for 3 days, and his condition improves. Tests performed include a chest x-ray, an EKG, and blood tests. The hospital receives $2100 from Medicaid. Based on an FFS payment schedule, the actual cost of Mr. Holland's stay is $1700.

reimbursement with the per diem method of payment often conduct utilization review for the same reason.

Payment per episode of hospitalization

An example of *per-episode* payments include DRGs. These payments are a form of reimbursement developed by the Health Care Financing Administration (HCFA) for Medicare reimbursement of acute hospital care. DRGs are based on a classification system that uses patient diagnosis to determine the amount of payment to a hospital from Medicare.

The risk of financial loss is as prevalent with DRG payments as it is with per diem payments. Medicare is at risk for the number of admissions, while the hospital is at risk for the length of hospital stay and the resources used during the hospital stay. The sooner a patient is discharged, the less money the hospital spends on treating the patient. Whether the patient is discharged to his or her home or to another level of care does not matter because regardless of where the patient goes after the acute episode, the hospital is reimbursed the same amount.

As a result of per-episode payment, the focus of acute health care providers has been to stabilize patients quickly and discharge them to a lower level of care as soon as possible, thus creating reduced lengths of stay in hospitals. This is done in hopes of generating a profit at the acute level. The potential of financial loss remains, however, if the hospital provider is not efficient and the patient stays in the hospital too long. Consider the scenario on Page 31.

Mrs. Taylor is an 82-year-old who fell and fractured her hip. She required an open reduction internal fixation and stayed in the hospital 6 days post-surgery. The cost of her hospital stay was $20,000. On the basis of the hip/femur procedure's DRG, Medicare reimbursed the hospital $12,000.

Today, patients are being discharged sooner and sicker than ever before, creating the need for less intensive sub-acute facilities, such as outpatient rehabilitation or skilled nursing facilities. In fact, growth in the sub-acute market has increased over the past several years as a result of cost-containment efforts.[14] Consider the course of Mrs. Taylor's rehabilitation:

Because Mrs. Taylor lives alone and requires moderate assistance with transfers and gait, she was discharged from the hospital to a local skilled nursing facility. Here, she was able to receive occupational and physical therapy two times per day, 7 days per week. She remained in this facility for 2 weeks and was discharged home after becoming independent in her activities of daily living, transfers, and ambulation.

The DRG prospective payment system has been criticized because it does not account for differing patients' clinical attributes. People whose care is more costly due to the nature of their disabilities are at risk of not receiving the services they require, according to Margaret G. Stineman, MD, Associate Professor in Rehabilitation Medicine at the University of Pennsylvania Medical Center, Philadelphia. Stineman is currently working on a project funded by the National Institutes of Health that focuses on improving quality and determining equitable hospital payment through the Functional Independence Measure—Function Related Groups (FIM-FRGs). This project puts patients into one of 20 diagnostic categories, such as stroke or spinal cord injury, and further separates these patients by severity of disability and age at admission to rehabilitation.[15]

Another per-diem payment method is anticipated for Medicare's prospective payment system for outpatient care. The Balanced Budget Act of 1997 mandated that an arbitrary cap of $1500 be placed on outpatient facilities receiving Medicare reimbursement beginning January 1, 1999. By January 2001, a new prospective payment system will be proposed by the Secretary of Health and Human Services to Congress to replace the cap with a new PPS. This reimbursement system is to be based on the classification of individuals by diagnostic category and prior use of services in both inpatient and outpatient settings.[7] As a result, HCFA has funded the development of *ambulatory patient groups (APGs)* with plans to use them as the basis for the outpatient prospective payment system.[16]

Payment per patient

Payment per patient, or capitation, is a common method of payment with HMOs. Under capitation, the hospital bears all the risk of financial loss (ie, through the number of admissions, lengths of stay, and resources used). In this situation, it is the hospital staff who performs utilization review to make sure that each admission, treatment, and hospital day is justified.

The following two scenarios offer an example of how capitation puts the provider at risk:

> *Laurie is enrolled in Healthy Care HMO, which contracts with St. Peter's Hospital. The hospital receives $20 per month as a capitation fee from Healthy Care. During the 5 years that Laurie is enrolled in Healthy Care, she remains healthy and does not set foot in the hospital. St. Peter's Hospital is paid $1200 even though no intervention was performed.*
>
> *Michelle has been enrolled in Healthy Care HMO for the past 5 years. In the course of that time, she has developed back pain that is so severe she requires a laminectomy and fusion. The hospital receives $20 per month as her capitated fee, which adds up to $1200 for the 5 years she has been enrolled in Healthy Care HMO. Her surgical and postoperative care cost $18,000.*

With capitation, the health of the enrolled subscribers often influences the provider's profit or loss. In the two examples above, we can see that the healthy enrollee, Laurie, required no care and the provider realized a profit. One the other hand, Michelle, the patient requiring surgical intervention, used $18,000 worth of health care, causing the provider to lose $16,800. In this case, the provider would essentially need to enroll 14 healthy members like Laurie (who required no care) to balance Michelle's costs.

Payment per institution (global budget)

Global budgets are used in Veterans Affairs (VA) hospitals and some staff-model HMOs (ie, the Kaiser Permanente system hospitals). It is also a common method of payment in Canada and many European nations. The VA hospitals are paid one fixed sum annually by the government, which is financed through federal income taxes. Similarly, the Kaiser Health Plan pays its hospitals a fixed amount each year, which is financed by large numbers of enrollees. Physicians, nurses, allied health professionals employed by the hospital, as well as laboratory technicians, custodians, and other personnel are all paid out of this global budget.

This form of payment is considered the most bundled because no matter how many expensive tests and services are provided, the hospital is forced to operate within its annual budget. The following scenario illustrates how there are no bills generated or payments made from outside insurance companies when there is a global budget in place:

> *Grayson Struthers, a member of a prominent staff-model HMO plan, has a sudden onset of dizziness, loss of appetite, weakness, and headache over a week's time. He goes to the hospital for evaluation and is admitted with a severely low hemoglobin count. After several tests and diagnostic procedures, it is found that Grayson has colon cancer. He has surgery to resect the cancer and undergoes a colostomy. Postoperatively, he develops gastro-intestinal bleeding from another site. His condition deteriorates over a 2-week period, and he lapses into a coma and dies. No hospital bill is generated as a result of Mr. Struthers' admission, and no payments are made from any insurance company to the hospital for his care.*

PHYSICAL THERAPY REIMBURSEMENT

Although FFS reimbursement is still used today to pay for physical therapy services, fewer than 9% of reimbursement cases fall under this payment system[17] in areas of the country where managed health care is more prevalent. Managed health care changes have catalyzed an increase in bundled payment methods (DRGs, per diem, and capitated payments), shifting financial risk from the insurer to the provider. As a result, physical therapy has shifted from being a revenue-generating center to a cost center that dips into the dwindling pot of bundled payments.

Physical therapy is reimbursed in different ways, depending on the payer, the type of services provided, and the site and level of care at which the services were provided. For example, if patients with Medicare coverage make up the majority of an acute hospital's inpatient population, then prospective payment by the DRG system would be expected. Inpatient physical therapy is typically paid for from the funds the hospital receives from these per-episode rates. In contrast, if the physical therapist sees many outpatients who are members of HMOs, then the reimbursement method will likely be per visit (with a limited frequency or duration policy set by the payer) or by capitation.

Who decides which method of reimbursement will be instituted? Typically, the payer determines the type of payment method when negotiating contracts with hospitals and outpatient facilities.[10] However, if there is an opportunity for input into this decision, the provider/facility should assess its needs or "personality" for compatibility with the available options. Consider how knowing the "personality" of your facility is beneficial in the following scenario:

> *Your private outpatient physical therapy facility is negotiating with a managed care organization (MCO), Rain-or-Shine Health Care, for a contract. As part-owner of this facility, you have been invited to offer input into how payments will be made. In preparation, you have considered the "personality" of your facility and its ability to adapt to new payment methods. Your facility's intense, short-duration treatment plans are a clue that your facility would not want a per-visit method of reimbursement because this method would limit the reimbursement for each visit. Because you have a relatively small practice, you sense you would not generate enough revenue with capitation (PMPM payments) to keep your practice viable. Furthermore, you consider that fee-for-service reimbursement is out of the question with this MCO. Instead, you decide to lobby for a per-episode method of payment, which would allow your facility to benefit from your efficiency—the fact that your patients have fewer visits.*

Inpatient Physical Therapy Reimbursement Issues

In the past, FFS payments were based on the UCR system. However, because many providers failed to be efficient, this system of payment became a major factor in rapidly rising health care costs.

Medicare dealt with this issue during the mid-1980s when it developed its PPS, using patients' DRGs as the basis for payment for acute inpatient care. The PPS is a fee schedule that sets pre-determined payments for hospital services regardless of the actual expenses to treat the patient. Two changes that DRGs brought about include the following:

1. A major reduction of inpatient physical therapy revenue from Medicare.
2. An overall decrease in the hospital's Medicare revenue.

Of Medicare's 470 DRG classifications, only four allow specific reimbursement for physical therapy. These four classifications include the following:
- Major joint procedures
- Specific cardiovascular procedures excluding transient ischemic angina
- Hip/femur procedures
- Medical back problems

Approximately 45% of Medicare patients fall into one of these four physical therapy DRG classifications, which means that any reduction of these four categories will lead to a major reduction of inpatient physical therapy revenue from Medicare, in addition to an overall decrease in hospital-Medicare revenue. Because DRGs are a per-episode payment, physical therapists need to actually treat Medicare patients in order to generate income from Medicare.

Medicare typically does not increase its DRG rates to account fully for hospitals' added expenses, such as salaries for personnel in short supply, supplies to maintain universal precautions for all patients, and increasing costs of utilities. As a result, it becomes more and more difficult to offer competitive salaries to hospital clinicians without operating at a deficit.[18]

SKILLED NURSING FACILITY REIMBURSEMENT

In the Balanced Budget Act (BBA) of 1997, Congress mandated the development of a case mix-adjusted PPS to begin July 1, 1998, for all skilled nursing facility services. These services include physical therapy provided to patients covered by Medicare Part A. This PPS will be phased in over 4 years, including a transition period when part of the reimbursement will be determined by the facility and the rest determined by the federal rate. Currently, HCFA is developing a case-mix measure that can be used to ensure that a facility is paid sufficiently for the resources necessary to provide appropriate care. It is believed that Medicare will use version III of the Resource Utilization Groups System (RUGS-III) classification system.[19-21]

The American Physical Therapy Association (APTA) states these RUGS-III classifications will be based on the total number of minutes of therapy per week, days of therapy per week, and the number and types of therapy. Each rehabilitation group will be given a rehabilitation index based on the complexity of the patient and the amount of staff time that is devoted to residents in each group. Rates are determined based on the rehabilitation index multiplied by the cost of staff time. The more time and services a category requires, the larger the weight will be.[19]

Outpatient Reimbursement Issues

When inpatient physical therapy services began to experience the crunch of DRGs on reimbursement, more outpatient facilities were created to enhance revenue. Because DRGs only applied to inpatient care, and outpatient services had fewer restrictions, this was a reasonable strategy.

Over time, however, outpatient physical therapy has become less of a revenue enhancer. Payers began to realize that not all outpatient care is cheaper than inpatient care, nor has hospital-based outpatient care been the cheapest way to obtain care. As a result, restrictions have emerged, limiting both coverage of and payment for outpatient physical therapy services.

Three types of outpatient coverage restrictions have come about in physical therapy:

1. Coverage limited to outpatient facilities that meet certain criteria, such as facilities that contract with specific HMOs.
2. Limits placed on the frequency, duration, or types of services provided and a cap on the total payment allowed.
3. Monitoring, on a case-by-case basis, the necessity of physical therapy through requiring prior approval and post-treatment utilization review of insurance claims.

The more popular payment methods for outpatient services include capitation and its variation—the payment of a fraction of the program's costs or charges up to a predetermined maximum. For example, after services have been provided, Medicare intermediaries review the case to determine if care was necessary and reasonable. If care was justified and the patient's yearly deductible allowance has been previously paid, then 80% of the allowed charge is paid to the provider. The additional 20% comes directly from the patient in the form of a copayment.

A fourth restriction is yet to be placed on outpatient physical therapy services as a result of the 1997 BBA. The BBA established a $1500 cap per beneficiary on outpatient rehabilitation services (including physical therapy and speech pathology services) under Medicare Part B. Professional organizations are actively lobbying for the flexibility to evaluate individual patient needs in setting more reasonable limits.

MANAGING UNDER MANAGED CARE

As managed health care has implemented prospective payment systems and more bundled payment methods, we can see that physical therapy is not the revenue-generating center it once was when fee-for-service retrospective reimbursement prevailed. Under prospective payment, physical therapy operates as a cost center that taps into a dwindling pool of resources. It is now more important than ever to provide services in a more efficient and economical way. Following are some suggestions for managing under these managed care conditions.

Creating Profit

Managed care payment plans shift risk to the provider, making it increasingly difficult to keep costs within budget, much less to generate a profit. Therefore, in order to survive, strategies must be implemented to minimize losses and operate efficiently.

Profit can be realized by any combination of the following:
1. Increasing the volume of patients seen
2. Reducing patient costs by treating efficiently
3. Negotiating for high capitation rates[22,23]

Increase patient volume

To increase the volume of patients seen, there needs to be a high volume of referrals and enough payers to have a large patient base to serve. This becomes challenging when a facility offers limited services or has to compete with other providers for contracts.

Reduce patient costs

Reducing patient costs is paramount to break even or turn a profit. As payment methods become more bundled, efficient treatment of patients becomes essential. This will benefit providers because they won't be wasting their time treating someone eight times with treatment A when they should have discharged the patient after four visits using treatment B.

The most efficient and cost-effective ways to treat patients are being sought through outcomes research. *Efficiency* is the change in an outcome over time or how long it took to achieve the outcome. In contrast, *cost-effectiveness* measures the magnitude of change per unit of cost, or how much it costs to achieve the outcome.

Negotiating contracts

Negotiating with insurance companies is a tricky business because of competition with other providers for the same patients. If the bid is too high, the contract may be lost to lower bidding providers. If a provider's bid is too low, subsequent revenue may be insufficient to meet expenses, requiring a constant struggle to supply quality treatment and meet costs.

Create a "payer mix" that best meets your needs

It is important to have information on what types of payers are represented by patients in order to know the "payer mix." For example, if 10% of the patients are from insurance plans that pay by FFS, 35% are from HMOs, 35% are from PPOs, and 20% are from Medicare, the provider might break even. In contrast, if the Medicare patient load increases, expenses may exceed revenues.

Create new levels of care

Acute care services are very expensive, so it is advantageous to create subacute facilities to provide care for individuals needing less skilled care at a lower cost. For example, some larger hospitals have varying levels of care, such as intensive care units, acute floors, sub-acute floors, or long-term care wings. Other sub-acute levels of care include skilled nursing facilities, convalescent homes, assisted care living facilities, board and care facilities, home health services, and outpatient services.

Coping with Managed Care

Many critics of managed care have argued that poor quality treatments will result from the inverse relationship between cost and profit. It seems nearly impossible to provide comparable quality care in less time and for less pay. Some fear that provider-patient relationships will be threatened through managed competition and argue that health care reform should be implemented to preserve continuity of care.[24,25]

Furthermore, the restrictions that managed care has created (ie, cost-containment strategies, shorter lengths of stays, strict utilization review) have forced smaller, private practice facilities to join with larger practices or networks. These changes may be quite discouraging if we maintain the pre-managed care mindset that quality care means being paid more to provide more.

No matter how bleak the outlook of managed care, we must note the many positive characteristics that our current health care environment offers. Particularly because it is inevitable that we will be operating in a managed care environment, we must, therefore, remain open-minded, flexible, and creative as we practice our profession.

Managed care keeps providers in check, while at the same time controlling utilization and quality care. Some benefits reaped from managed competition include the following:

Efficiency

With more bundled payments, providers are forced to become more efficient to keep their costs down. Clinical pathways set standards that aid clinicians to progress in an expedient manner. Database studies and outcomes research can help identify more efficient protocols and aid in decision making.

Cost effectiveness

With limited treatment sessions and visits, providers are forced to use more cost-effective treatments. Less costly but equally effective methods of treatment, such as group treatment and patient education, must be evaluated.

Ethical and legal issues

To successfully compete for health care contracts, it is imperative that providers practice within ethical and legal constraints. Managed competition compels providers to maintain ethical standards. By doing this, providers should be evaluated more favorably by consumers (payers and patients) and, therefore, be more likely to receive contracts and referrals.

Accountability

Through utilization review and utilization management, outcomes research, and practice profiles, providers are now more accountable for the quality of their care (see Chapter 12). By using such systems, providers, patients, and payers all benefit.

Practice profile

Those providers who improve or maintain an outstanding practice profile, based on outcomes data, will be at an advantage when renewing or negotiating new contracts. Furthermore, individual providers can analyze their own practice profile, compare themselves with other providers, and identify areas that need improvement.

Refer to other providers

It is advantageous to refer a patient to an appropriate outside provider when it is not possible for the original provider to treat him or her effectively and efficiently. This not only benefits the patient, but it also saves time and money on cases that a provider is not equipped to handle. For example, a patient comes into a sports medicine clinic with a diagnosis of left cerebrovascular accident with right hemiparesis. Because the clinic is too busy to spend more than 15 to 20 minutes with each patient and is not equipped with proper equipment or knowledgeable staff, it would be wise to refer the patient to an outpatient neurological rehabilitation center. This benefits the patient by enhancing the quality of service provided and prevents the sports clinic from wasting time trying to attempt treatment it does not routinely provide.

Autonomy

Managed care allows providers to maintain more autonomy than possible under the more traditional FFS reimbursement structure. Under an FFS payment method, the provider may be limited as to what services the insurance company will cover. Capitation, in contrast, allows the provider the freedom to determine treatment alternatives. It is up to the provider to decide what treatment methods will provide the most efficient and cost-effective outcomes.

These aspects of managed care enhance, rather than hinder, the quality of care we can provide as physical therapists. If we as professionals are to survive in this new environment, we must appreciate the opportunities that managed care brings about.

SUMMARY

Health Care Financing

Financing is the flow of money from individuals and/or employers to the health plan, whereas *reimbursement* is the flow of money from the payer (health plan) to the provider. *Retrospective* and *prospective payment systems* differ in the relative risk to payer and provider. *Bundling* is a description of the volume of services the provider delivers for a given payment. *Risk* is the potential for a provider to lose money, earn less money, or spend more time without additional payment on a reimbursement transaction.

The financing of health care in the United States has been accomplished via four methods: out-of-pocket payments, individual private insurance, employment-based private insurance, and government-financed health insurance.

Out-of-pocket payment involves a single, direct payment from the individual seeking medical care to the one providing the care. Because health care in this country is considered a right and not a privilege, people do not purchase health care as they would a luxury item. Because it is impossible to predict how much medical care will be needed in a lifetime, this payment method is no longer realistic, as most people are unable to pay today's immense medical bills.

Individual private insurance involves two transactions: a payment from the individual enrollee to the insurer and a payment from the insurer to the provider. A list of providers and services that are covered by the insurer is usually provided with the stipulation that the enrollee pay a deductible, a copayment, and/or pay for services not covered by the plan.

Employment-based private insurance is employer-financed health care. As a fringe benefit of employment, employee health care premiums are paid for in full or in part by employers. Premiums for these health care plans can be based on experience rating or community rating. *Experience rating* involves the classification of groups of prospective subscribers into various utilization levels, thereby discriminating between healthy and less healthy groups of people. *Community rating* premiums are based on human need and do not discriminate between groups of people.

Government-financed health care programs, administered through Medicare and Medicaid, are financed by taxpayers. Medicare uses public funds and monthly premiums to finance hospital insurance (Medicare A) and physician/outpatient services (Medicare B) for the elderly. Medicare C is a new addition to Medicare that offers its enrollees a choice of health plans. Medicaid uses public funds to finance medical assistance to the poor. Although government-financed health insurance has improved access to health care for the poor and elderly, it has aggravated the problem of rising costs. A growing need for assistance parallels growing health care costs. Unemployment, high health care costs, a growing elderly population, and increased lifespan of those with chronic conditions are just a few of the issues that complicate the need for these government-assisted plans.

Health Care Reimbursement

Four basic types of managed care reimbursement patterns exist in the United States. They vary in their level of bundled services and financial risk: *fee-for-service payments, per-visit payments, per-episode payments, and capitation*. Three forms of managed care that use these reimbursement methods include *fee-for-service reimbursement with utilization review, preferred provider organizations*, and *health maintenance organizations*.

Physician payments can be via *fee for service, per visit, per episode*, or *per patient (capitation)*. Hospitals are reimbursed either *per procedure, per diem, per episode, per patient (capitation)*, or through a *global budget*. Physical therapy is considered a *cost center* and is reimbursed either through *fee for service, per episode, per diem*, or *capitation*. In all cases, managed care tends to favor the more bundled reimbursement methods of a prospective payment system that places more risk on the providers.

Coverage restrictions have recently come about to further control utilization. Restrictions on outpatient physical therapy include reimbursing preferred providers only, limiting the number of services or visits or maximum reimbursement, and defining "medical necessity" on a case-by-case basis.

Strategies necessary to survive in the world of managed care require action that limits costs and increases efficiency. It is wise to recognize that although managed care appears to threaten quality care, it can actually enhance quality via improved efficiency and cost effectiveness, monitoring ethical standards and encouraging accountability, improving practice profiles, and encouraging referrals of patients to other providers when necessary.

REFERENCES

1. Bodenheimer TS, Grumbach K. *Understanding Health Policy—A Clinical Approach.* Stamford, Conn: Appleton and Lange; 1995.
2. *1996 Current Population Survey.* US Bureau of the Census, March, 1996. hhs-info@census.gov (or call 301-457-3242).
3. Stewart DL, Abeln SH. *Documenting Functional Outcomes in Physical Therapy.* St. Louis, MO: Mosby-Year Book, Inc.; 1993.
4. Newhouse JP, Manning WG, Morris CN, et al. Some interim results from a controlled trial of cost sharing in health insurance. *N Engl J Med.* 1981;305(25):1501-1507.
5. Relman AS. Assessment and accountability: the third revolution in medical care. *N Engl J Med.* 1988;319(18):1220-1222.
6. *Frequently Asked Questions.* New York, NY: GHI (Group Health Insurance); http://www.ghi-medicare.com/bene/faq.html. 4/26/98.
7. *The Balanced Budget Act: How it Affects Physical Therapy,* Alexandria, Va: American Physical Therapy Association; http://www.apta.org/govt_aff/bbasynop.html. 4/26/98.
8. *Questions and Answers to Provisions of the Balanced Budget Act.* Alexandria, Va: American Physical Therapy Association; http://www.apta.org/govt_aff/bbaq&a.html. 4/26/98.
9. Hoffman C, Rice D, Sung HY. Persons with chronic conditions; their prevalence and costs. *JAMA.* 1996;276(18):1473-1479.
10. Nugent J. Payment methods under managed care. *PT-Magazine of Physical Therapy.* 1995;3(9):34-36.
11. Cohn R. Managed care in intermediate settings part II: selection and implementation of a contract. *PT-Magazine of Physical Therapy.* 1996;4(9):20, 23.
12. Welch WP, Hillman AL, Pauly MV. Toward new technologies for HMOs. *Milbank Q.* 1990;68:21.
13. Kerr EA, Mittman BS, Hays RD, Siu AL, Leake B, Brook RH. Managed care and capitation in California: How do physicians at financial risk control their own utilization? *Ann Intern Med.* 1995;123(7):500-504.
14. Cohn R. Managed care in intermediate care settings part 1: Implications and strategies. *PT-Magazine of Physical Therapy.* 1996;4(7):28, 31.
15. Kaminski C. Renaissance doctor: Margaret Stineman's art of healing. *Advance for Directors in Rehabilitation.* 1998;7(4):90.
16. *APG Essentials.* Cleveland, OH: ORION Consulting, Inc. http://www.orion-consulting.com/apg/#whatarepags. 3/25/98.
17. Schroffel B, CEO, UCSF Medical Center. *Questions and Challenges for Physical Therapists in an Ever-loving Managed Care Marketplace,* presented at California Chapter Conference, American Physical Therapy Association, Burlingame, Calif. October 26, 1996.

18. Rasmussen B. Reimbursement and hospital physical therapy. *Clinical Management in Physical Therapy.* 1990;10(6):15-17.
19. APTA. Skilled nursing facilities will be reimbursed under Medicare prospective payment system beginning July 1. *Iowa Recap: quarterly newsletter of the Iowa Physical Therapy Association & Foundation.* 1998: 5.
20. *Synopsis—Prospective Payment System and Consolidated Billing Regulations for Skilled Nursing Homes.* Alexandria, VA: American Physical Therapy Association; http://www.apta.org/govt_aff/pps.html. 4/6/98.
21. Balanced Budget Agreement signed into law—Significant changes ahead for Medicare. in *Regulatory Matters,* August, *1997,* Alexandria, VA: American Physical Therapy Association; http://www.apta.org/govt_aff/jan_reg_update.html. 4/6/98.
22. Rasmussen B. Capitated reimbursement rates for the office-based PT. *PT-Magazine of Physical Therapy.* 1993;42-46.
23. Finkler SA. Capitated hospital contract: the empty beds versus filled beds controversy. *Health Care Manage Rev.* 1995;20(3):88-91.
24. Emanuel EJ, Brett AS. Managed Competition and the patient-physician relationship. *N Engl J Med.* 1993;329(12):879-882.
25. Clancy CM, Himmelstein DU, Woolhandler S. Questions and answers about managed competition. *Int J Health Serv.* 1993;23(2):213-218.

TEST YOUR SKILLS

1. What is/are the concerns (advantages, disadvantages, incentives, and risks) for payers, providers, and patients under each reimbursement system?

	Payer concerns	Provider concerns	Patient concerns
Fee-for-service (FFS)			
PPO (reduced FFS)			
Per diem			
Per episode			
Capitation			

CHECK YOUR RESPONSES

	Payer concerns	Provider concerns	Patient concerns
Fee-for-service (FFS)	•Higher cost of insurance premiums •Incentive to enroll high numbers of low-risk subscribers •Incentive to limit number of covered services in the policy •Incentive to review cases to justify payment	•Increased volume of services results in increased revenue •Increased number# of visits or length of stay results in increased revenue •Increased volume of patients results in increased revenue •Incentive to work less efficiently and over bill	•Freedom of choice to seek medical care from any provider •May have to pay a higher premium or higher out-of-pocket costs •Covered services may be limited by payer •At risk of receiving minimal services and being billed excessively
PPO (reduced FFS)	•Incentive to enroll high numbers of low-risk subscribers •Incentive to limit number of covered services in the policy •Contract with providers who agree to accept the lowest FFS fee schedule	Incentives to: •Reduce time spent with each patient •Increase volume of patients or visits; •Increase volume of less labor-intensive services •Be more time efficient •Delegate treatment to lower-cost support personnel	•Lower premium and out-of-pocket costs than in FFS plans •Less freedom of choice to select provider •May have to pay a higher premium or higher out- of- pocket costs if provider is not in PPO group •Covered services may be limited by payer
Per diem	•Incentive to enroll high numbers of low-risk subscribers •Incentive to limit number of covered days in the policy •Shifts part of risk to the provider as payer liability is limited at a per-diem rate (usually for hospitalization)	Incentives to: •Limit number of services performed each day, especially expensive ones •Maximize patient's length of stay if revenue is greater than costs to provide care •Delegate treatment to lower lower-cost support personnel	•Lower premium and out-of-pocket costs (is often enrolled in a PPO or HMO) •Less freedom of choice to select provider •May have to pay a higher premium or higher out of pocket costs if provider is not in designated group
Per episode	•Incentive to enroll high numbers of low-risk subscribers •Incentive to limit covered diagnoses and set low limits on certain diagnostic groups. •Shifts part of risk to provider as payer liability is limited to a set maximum per episode of care	Incentives to: •Maximize volume of admissions or patient referrals •Limit number of services performed each day, especially expensive ones •Delegate treatment to lower cost support personnel •Decrease length of stay or duration of treatments (high turnover) •Refer elsewhere or transfer to another level of care	•Lower premium and out-of-pocket costs (is often enrolled in Medicare or HMO) •Less freedom of choice to select provider •May have to pay a higher premium or higher out- of- pocket costs if provider is not in designated group •At risk of under under-treatment, early discharge, and transfer to another level of care to reduce provider risk

	Payer concerns	**Provider concerns**	**Patient concerns**
Capitation	•Incentive to enroll high numbers of low- risk subscribers •Shifts most of risk to provider as payer liability is limited to a set capitation rate (per member per month)	Incentives to •Prevent hospitalization and high-cost illnesses •Limit number of visits and treatments •Push for early discharge •Be efficient with provision of care; •Maximize number of healthy patients enrolled in contracted groups	•Lower premium and out-of-pocket costs (is often enrolled in HMO) •Less freedom of choice to select provider •May have to pay a higher premium or higher out-of-pocket costs if provider is not in designated group •At risk of undertreatment, early discharge, and transfer to another level of care to reduce provider risk

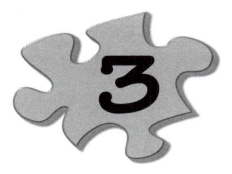

COST-CONTAINMENT STRATEGIES

Wendy Kristy, MPT

CONTROLLING THE HIGH COST OF HEALTH CARE

This chapter discusses current types of cost controls in the US health care system. Cost controls can be applied to both the financing and reimbursement components of health care spending and are used in an effort to decrease overall spending, or flow of money in health care (Figure 3.1).[1]

Growing Populations and Expanding Costs

Increased access to health care and technology has led to the need for cost containment. Historically, the expansion of medical services occurred during a time in American history when there was no national debt or inflation. This resulted in an increase in access to health care, technology, and specialization, and culminated in the enactment of government-subsidized health care (Medicare and Medicaid). Inflation began shortly afterward, causing health care costs to sky-rocket, contributing to a growing national debt. Hence, the "era of cost containment" ensued.

Today, the need for cost containment remains, as health care costs continue to rise in the presence of a growing need for medical services. The chronically ill and growing elderly populations are two examples of groups who have high needs for medical services. The number of people with chronic health

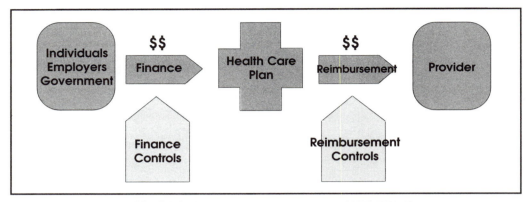

FIGURE 3.1 *Cost-control strategies. Adapted with permission from Bodenheimer TS, Grumbach K.* Understanding Health Policy: A Clinical Approach. *Norwalk, Conn: Appleton & Lange; 1995.*

conditions is growing rapidly due to advanced medical technology and decreased mortality from infectious diseases.[2] Also, as the fastest growing population in America, the aging baby boomers will inherently require more medical care than other age groups.

Chronic conditions

According to a report by the Robert Wood Johnson Foundation, nearly 100 million Americans have chronic conditions that place limitations on daily activities. These conditions are major causes of illness, disability, and death. The annual cost to care for these people is $475 billion and is predicted to double by the year 2050.[2] High costs for people with chronic care needs are due in part to a need for a broad scope of social, community, and personal services, as well as medical and rehabilitative care. As the number of people with chronic conditions grows, the demand on physical therapists, physicians, allied health professionals, and support groups will also grow dramatically in the years ahead.[3]

Chronic conditions affect people of all types and ages.[3,4] Medical care for those with chronic ailments accounts for the largest share of the nation's health care bill, amounting to three-quarters of the direct costs of physicians, therapists, and hospitals (Figure 3.2).[3]

Surprisingly, the majority of people with chronic conditions are not the elderly. Although the elderly are the fastest growing population in the United States (80% of whom have at least one chronic illness), this group makes up only one-fourth of the population with chronic conditions.

Because people with chronic conditions have greater health needs at any age, their costs are disproportionately higher. It is estimated that this popula-

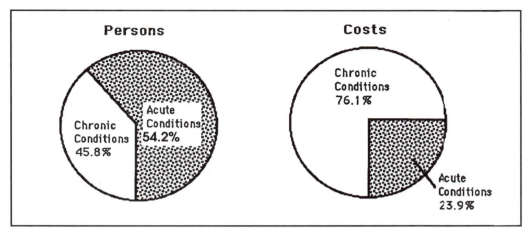

Persons

Costs

FIGURE 3.2 *Prevalence of acute and chronic conditions and related health care costs. While less than half of the population reported chronic conditions, they accounted for more than 75% of direct medical care costs in the United States in 1987.[2]*

tion is at greater risk for being under-insured, has higher rates of utilization, and has higher health care costs.[3] Because people are living longer, even with chronic diseases, we can expect even greater health care expenditures for the chronically ill in the future.

According to Hoffman, et al, nearly half the population is living with a chronic disease or impairment that is incurable.[2] For this reason, it is thought that every American family is likely to be caring for at least one family member with a chronic condition. However, family size is shrinking, leaving fewer members available to provide help to those members who need care. This places more of a burden on the American health care system and is a major source of health care costs.

The expanding elderly population

The growing elderly population will also place a burden on the health care industry due to its increased need for medical services (Figure 3.3). As mentioned before, 80% of this population have a chronic disorder, and 44% percent of them have more than one condition.[3] Currently, informal caregivers (unpaid family, friends, and community volunteers) provide much of the care to this population. Because family sizes are shrinking, there will be fewer caregivers for a growing elderly population.[2] This will undoubtedly increase the need for home health medical services and contribute to further rising costs in health care.

Consider the growing number of elderly people with Alzheimer's disease. Research shows that one in 10 people older than 65 years and 50% of those

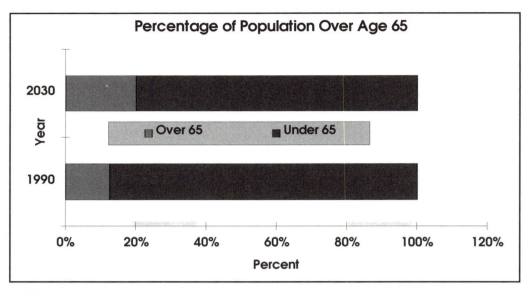

FIGURE 3.3 *One in eight persons was over the age of 65 in 1990. By 2030, one in five persons will be over the age of 65. Source: Day JC. Population Projections of the United States by Age, Sex, Race, and Hispanic Origin: 1993-2050. Washington, DC: US Bureau of Census; 1993. Current Population Reports. Series P-25, No. 1104.*

older than 80 years have the disease today. The cost of a person with Alzheimer's disease averages $7682, 70% higher than the annual average of $4524 for other Medicare beneficiaries. By itself, Alzheimer's disease comprises $100 billion a year in health care costs.[5]

Future needs for health care will continue to grow, inevitably increasing our nation's health care costs. As it is, the demand for health care is surpassing the financial resources most individuals have to pay for it. Therefore, methods of cost containment must be devised to prevent further increases in health care costs while maintaining quality of care.

FINANCING CONTROLS

Cost controls can be applied to either or both the financing or reimbursement aspects of health care.[1,6] With financing controls, it is thought that by limiting the funding for health care (financing), we simultaneously limit the spending on health care (reimbursement). Two types of financing control strategies include *regulation* and *competition.*

Regulation

Regulation strategies are attempts by the government to decrease, or control, the amount of money that is paid into a health plan. When insurance is financed with taxpayer money, such as Medicare, there needs to be congressional approval to increase or decrease taxes paid toward health care. Current political issues are focused on limiting Medicare and Medicaid financing. Tax cuts directed toward health care would directly affect Medicare by limiting the amount of money available to spend on public assistance for health care. Regulation of health insurance premiums would restrict third-party payer spending by limiting funds available for reimbursement. Consider the following example of government regulation:

In a democratic country where government regulates health care, congress passes a health care bill that limits health care premiums to a 4% annual increase. Because the premiums finance health care plans throughout this country, providers (physicians, hospitals, physical therapists, etc) are also limited to a 4% increase per year.[1]

Competition

Another attempt at decreasing health care financing involves competitive strategies, also known as *managed competition*. Managed competition occurs when health insurance plans compete with each other for enrollees. This strategy attempts to prevent employment-based private insurance plans from driving up health care costs. Unfortunately, two barriers have prevented effective competition:

1. The lack of cost-conscious consumers
2. Private third-party payers competing for low-risk (which means lower cost) groups of enrollees

Cost Consciousness

When an individual pays out-of-pocket for his or her health care, he or she becomes acutely aware of the cost and, thereby, becomes a conscientious consumer. When employers pay for health insurance premiums, the individual employees are insulated from the cost and may not become "cost conscious." Some policy makers believe that those recipients, who do not bear any financial responsibility for their health care, tend to over-use medical services, which drives up health care costs.[1,7,8]

Employers have found it advantageous to pay for their employees' health insurance because money spent on worker health care benefits is tax exempt. Employees are at a disadvantage when they pay directly for their health care insurance because they must first pay taxes on their income before it is used to pay for their health care. To shift a portion of the burden to consumers, some health care plans require employees (subscribers) to pay a percentage of the premium, a *deductible*, and/or a *copayment*.

Medical savings accounts (MSAs) have recently emerged as a strategy to increase consumer cost consciousness. This involves employers purchasing cheaper health plans with high deductibles for employees who choose to participate. The annual price difference between the highest priced health plan offered and the cheaper health plan purchased is put into a medical savings account. This money is then used by the employee toward the deductible and prescriptions not covered by the purchased plan. Whatever money is left in the account at the end of the year is retained by the employee. Advocates of MSAs say this strategy promotes cost consciousness by creating a situation in which, unless someone in your family fell very ill, every penny you spent on health care would be money you could have kept, saved, or spent on something else.[9]

In 1996, the RAND corporation studied the MSA approach to health care spending reduction. It projected that if everyone switched their health care plan to a high-deductible MSA plan, health care expenditures would decline by between 6% and 13%. However, the researchers admitted it is unlikely that everyone would switch from their current health plan to an MSA health plan. Realistically, this study concluded that the overall effect of offering MSAs as an option to other health care plans would result in minimal reduction of health care spending at best.[10]

Competing for Low-Risk Subscribers

Rather than competing on the basis of efficiency and quality of health care delivery, private insurance companies have competed for low-risk subscribers by offering them enticing health care plans. Because low-risk groups do not require expensive health care, as do higher risk groups, they have lower health care expenditures. Therefore, the goal of competition has become an issue of attracting large numbers of healthy enrollees. Such health plans profit when they collect premiums from healthy subscribers who do not use the medical services offered.

It is unlikely that any insurance company will be able to enroll only healthy people. More typically, a mix of both high- and low-risk groups are enrolled in health care plans. As a result, insurance companies have raised their premiums in order to cover the costs of providing care for their higher risk enrollees.

Summary of Financing Controls

It has been thought that health care costs can be decreased via the previously discussed financing controls: regulation, competition, raising consumer awareness of cost, and enrolling large numbers of low-risk groups. Analysts feel, however, that finance controls are weaker strategies than reimbursement controls. No matter what strategies are used to keep the financing side of the equation down, the reimbursement side remains untouched. If providers demand more reimbursement than is allowed through financing, a deficit occurs, and taxes/premiums ultimately need to be increased. Therefore, to control costs, we need to especially focus on controlling reimbursement.

REIMBURSEMENT CONTROLS

Cost-control strategies are also applied to the reimbursement side of health care payments (see Figure 3.1) and focus on the price and utilization of health care services. Similar to financing controls, *price controls* use both regulation and competition as cost-control strategies; whereas *utilization controls* use *bundled payments, cost sharing, utilization management*, and *supply limits* as cost-control strategies.

Price Controls

Price controls typically involve fee schedules, which are specified charges for specific medical services. Price controls come in two forms: *regulation* and *competition*.

Regulation

Medicare's payment system is an example of price controls using *regulation*. Prior to the mid 1980s, government-subsidized health care (Medicare, Medicaid) reimbursed health care providers using the UCR (usual, customary, and reasonable) physician fee screen. Here, the providers determined the charges for their services according to what they felt were UCR criteria. Since the mid 1980s, Medicare has implemented a prospective payment system (PPS) in which predetermined reimbursement rates are employed. An example of this is the diagnosis-related group (DRG) payment for acute hospitalization, in which reimbursement depends on a patient's diagnosis.[1,11] DRG rates are regulated by government agencies that act by legislative mandates.

More recently, the legislature passed the Balanced Budget Act (BBA) of 1997, which mandates that government-subsidized health care (Medicare) implement a PPS at other levels of care (ie, skilled nursing and home health).

The BBA has also established a controversial annual capitated fee payment of $1500 for outpatient rehabilitative services.[12] Currently, members of the American Physical Therapy Association have moved to repeal this $1500 limit, advocating that it will not cover the rehabilitation needs of those who encounter catastrophic/chronic problems (ie, stroke, traumatic brain injury).

Competition

Private insurance companies can use predetermined fee schedules to either regulate prices or to compete for lower provider fees. When fee schedules are determined by payers (insurance companies), they tend to be reduced-rate fees, which is a form of regulation. When fee schedules are determined by providers, *competition* occurs. Providers, with their own fee schedules, display their ability to provide care efficiently and cost effectively, hoping to secure a payer source and referrals.

There are two barriers that prevent price controls from successfully keeping costs down: *cost shifting* and *increased volume and intensity of services.*

Cost shifting

If a payer lowers the fee schedule for one hospital, that hospital will compensate by increasing its charges to other less restrictive payers. This is known as *cost shifting* and does not keep overall costs down. However, by implementing a uniform fee schedule for all payers, cost shifting cannot occur.[1]

Cape Town Physical Therapy contracts with a variety of payer sources that use different fee schedules. Payers A and B are private insurance companies that reimburse according to provider-based fee schedules. Payer C is an insurance company that reimburses according to its own fee schedule. Recently, Payer C lowered its fee schedule, meaning it now reimburses less for physical therapy services. This makes it difficult for Cape Town Physical Therapy to meet its own costs when treating patients insured by Payer C. In an effort to compensate for lost income from these patients, the facility decides to increase its charges on the fee schedules used for Payers A and B.

Increased volume and intensity of services

Although a uniform fee schedule will prevent cost shifting, it is often associated with an increase in the volume of patients seen and the number of services provided. This can be referred to as "patient churning," in which strict price controls encourage providers to compensate for lost income by increasing the use of their services.

Price controls appear to be a harmless form of cost control, but they are

Mercy Physical Therapy contracts with a variety of payer sources that all use a uniform fee schedule. In an effort to create more income, the facility enacts a policy that requires staff physical therapists to see no fewer than 14 patients in an 8-hour work day.

not problem-free. The use of uniform fee schedules allows some segments of the population access to health care they would otherwise not have. For example, Medicaid reimbursement rates have traditionally been very low, sometimes paying less than $0.25 on the dollar for charges for medically necessary treatments. As a result, Medicaid patients have difficulty finding providers who are willing to treat them.

Utilization Controls

The use of medical services, or *utilization*, is a measure of the number of health care services provided. Appropriate utilization has become an issue in the health care industry due to increased medical technology, training, and availability of health care services.[13] More advanced technology and an increase in the number of specialized physicians and services has led to an increase in use of expensive tests and procedures.[1,14] To curtail the rising costs associated with these procedures, four utilization controls have been implemented to help contain health care costs: *bundled payments, cost sharing, utilization management*, and *supply limits*.

Bundled payment methods

As discussed in Chapter 2, changing the unit of payment from the traditional fee-for-service (FFS) method to a more *bundled* payment method places financial risk on the provider. Providers who receive bundled payments are at risk of operating at a deficit. This was done to limit over-use of medical services and, therefore, decrease spending on health care. Bundled payment methods include *payment per visit, payment per episode*, and *capitation* (refer to Chapter 2 for definitions).

FFS payment methods are associated with an increase in utilization of services. Typically, patients are seen more frequently and have more services provided to them because providers do not have an incentive to be efficient (with their care). On the other hand, capitated payment methods create a different provider strategy: to keep patients healthy and out of the hospital and to limit services.

Patient cost sharing

Health care consumers become discouraged from over-using health care services when they become cost-conscious consumers. Through *patient cost sharing* at the point of service, consumers become aware of their health care costs and tend to not use services unless absolutely necessary. Cost sharing has been accomplished through imposing deductibles, copayments, and uncovered services (see Chapter 2). In contrast, full coverage leads to increased use per user of medical services.[1,7,8]

In a research project in which individuals were randomly placed into a variety of health care plans with varying degrees of cost sharing, it was found that cost sharing not only discouraged inappropriate use of health care services, but also discouraged cases in which health care was necessary and appropriate.[15] Consider the following scenario, which illustrates this point:

> *Janice Mackey underwent anterior cruciate ligament repair and was referred to a local physical therapist for follow-up care. When it was time to begin intensive physical therapy treatments, Janice thought that by the end of her rehabilitation, her $10 copayments would add up to nearly $300. She went to a few treatments before deciding to forego any further sessions and save her money. Four months later, she returned to her surgeon complaining of swelling and stiffness in her knee. After examining an MRI of Janice's knee, the surgeon concluded that she required arthroscopic surgery to release adhesions in her knee.*

Utilization management

Utilization management (UM) is an attempt to control costs, or spending, by discouraging inappropriate services. It involves pre-authorization of care, justification for care, and identification of a patient's readiness for discharge. Whereas *utilization review (UR)* is a retrospective review of clinical services already provided, UM is a prospective and concurrent review of medical services being provided.[16] Both UR and UM are connected to reimbursement because reimbursement may be denied if care is not justified.

Pre-authorization involves contacting the payer source prior to rendering services. This verifies that the patient has insurance coverage and that the payer is inclined to reimburse for necessary care. If a patient is in a setting where the provider is at risk (ie, bundled form of reimbursement), then the provider should review the case to justify current or continued care and identify the patient's readiness for discharge. If a UM firm is reviewing a case that requires justification for further treatment, the physician/provider will call the UM firm at set intervals to negotiate further care.

Typically, whoever is at financial risk will perform UM. For example, if the reimbursement is by capitation, it is to the provider's advantage to perform UM. This is done to prevent inappropriate services and over-extension of resources. If the reimbursement is FFS, it is in the payer's best interest to perform UM. If the reimbursement is per diem, then both the payer and the provider might perform UM. In this case, the payer would verify that care is justified and reasonable. Similarly, there is a financial incentive for the provider to discharge the patient to the next level of care as quickly as possible.

Another approach to UM includes *practice profiling*. This is an attempt to identify providers whose services, or patient outcomes, significantly deviate from those of other providers (for example, hospitals that have a higher than average re-admission rate). This approach can be used to identify providers who need intervention such as education or monitoring. Practice profiling has also been used to identify providers with efficient practice patterns and can be effective for use in contract negotiations.

Limiting health care supply/services

Limiting the number of specialized providers or services in a geographical area also reduces the cost of specialized services. This is known as *supply limits* and is a response to a phenomenon known as *supplier-induced demand*, in which the more services that are available creates a greater demand for those services. The use of magnetic resonance imaging (MRI) has followed this pattern. The greater number of MRI units that are available in a specific geographic area tends to be related to a greater demand for MRI diagnostic testing. On the other hand, when there are fewer MRI units available, there are fewer MRI tests ordered. With a supply limit on MRI availability, physicians are forced to prioritize their patients' need for this service based on urgency and appropriateness.[1]

The value of supply limits is yet to be fully understood. Wennberg and Gittelsohn have shown variations in geographical locations that demonstrate that use of medical services is related to the availability of those services.[18] Later research by Wennberg suggests that these differences are related to diversity of accepted opinions among physicians on the need and value of alternate treatments.[19] Research has also been done to evaluate the effect of limiting supply on outcomes, showing that the limitation of supplies (ie, intensive care beds) does not affect outcomes.[20] It has been speculated that health care providers (physicians) are better able to prioritize limited services based on appropriateness and urgency of need.

The following scenario illustrates how supply limits work. Specialized services are consolidated in one location and serve a general geographical region.

Randall Lacy is a World War II veteran who has been diagnosed with arteriosclerotic heart disease and requires bypass surgery. His doctor is a general practitioner, and there are no thoracic surgeons on staff. Recently, he has been experiencing unstable angina and is having to take nitroglycerin more frequently. His physician referred him to a thoracic surgeon in a major metropolitan center 180 miles from his home.

Mixed Controls

Managed care is truly a "melting pot" of cost-control strategies, with a combination of both financing and reimbursement cost-control mechanisms (Figure 3.4).

Typically, no single approach to cost containment is attempted without some other form of cost control co-existing with it. As well, there are common patterns of cost-control strategies among various managed care organizations. For example, *preferred provider organizations (PPOs)* often use utilization management, patient cost sharing, and price discounts on FFS fee schedules for provider reimbursement. *Individual practice association (IPA) HMOs* (see Chapter 2) use bundled payment methods in conjunction with a gatekeeper (a primary physician who manages the medical services of all patients under his or her care). On the other hand, *staff and group model HMOs* (see Chapter 2) use the most bundled payment methods (salaries and global budgets) (Table 3.1).

Recent Research Findings

To date, inconclusive evidence exists on whether or not cost-containment strategies are successful in decreasing overall health care costs or utilization. Nonetheless, these strategies are being used today, and health care providers who understand them are more effective and efficient in their practices. The following are a few examples of research conducted to explore the effects of cost-containment strategies in health care today.

We have discussed that DRG payments are associated with shorter lengths of stay. Kane, et al showed this was true in their 1987 research project that studied the impact of DRGs on inpatient rehabilitation.[21] (Note: shorter length of stay does not mean patients can get by with less health care, for when patients leave the hospital they do not necessarily return home. Rather, they enter a lower [cost] level of care, such as a skilled nursing facility, nursing home, receive home health care, or outpatient services.)

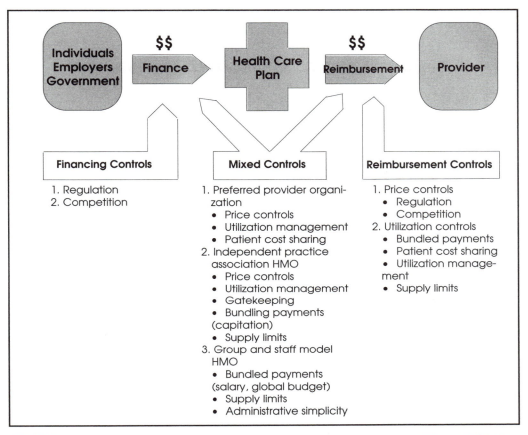

FIGURE 3.4 *The big picture of cost containment. A general overview of cost control in health care. Adapted with permission from Bodenheimer TS, Grumbach K.* Understanding Health Policy: A Clinical Approach. *Stamford, Conn: Appleton and Lange.*

Goldman, et al studied the effects of benefit design and managed care on health care costs of military health care beneficiaries. The comparison of government costs per adult beneficiary indicated that there were substantially higher costs with the use of the HMO-type health care plan than the traditional FFS plan. The authors attribute the HMO's higher per-beneficiary costs to reduced cost-sharing and lower out-of-pocket payments of the military beneficiaries.[22]

A 1989 study by Hillman, Pauly, and Kerstein compared hospitalization rates of patients covered by plans that used FFS, capitation, and salaried forms of reimbursement. They found that hospitalization rates of patients covered by HMO plans were lower than hospitalization rates of patients covered by FFS plans.[23]

A 1996 RAND study of Medicaid program spending determined that mem-

TABLE 3.1

Common cost-containment Strategies Used by Different Types of Managed Care Providers

Preferred Provider Organizations
- Price controls (discounted fee schedules determined by payers)
- Utilization management (pre-authorization, chart/case reviews, case managers)
- Patient cost sharing (copayments, deductibles, uncovered services)

Independent Practice Association HMOs
- Price controls (fee schedules)
- Utilization management (pre-authorization, chart/case reviews, case managers)
- Gatekeeping (use of a primary physician to manage each patient's care)
- Changing unit of payment to capitation (bundling payments)
- Regulating supply via selective contracting (contracting only with providers who are willing to provide services at discounted rates and who are efficient with outcomes)

Group and Staff Model HMOs
- Changing unit of payment to salary and global budgets (all providers are paid a salary, no fee schedules)
- Supply controls (more expensive and less used specialists are fewer in number and concentrated in a geographically strategic location)
- Administrative simplicity (because there is no third-party payer and all care is provided under one roof, there are fewer administrative steps)

Adapted from Bodenheimer TS, Grumbach K. Understanding Health Policy: A Clinical Approach. *Stamford, Conn: Appleton & Lange; 1995.*

ber utilization was successfully limited, resulting in significantly lower monthly health care expenditures for those recipients enrolled in HMOs as compared to those enrolled in FFS programs.[24]

According to Kerr, et al, physician groups that were reimbursed by capitation were influenced to devise their own management systems to contain costs. These groups have implemented utilization management methods, such as gatekeeping, pre-authorization, profiling, education, and guidelines to keep their costs down and profits up.[17]

These examples are a sampling of the current literature available on this extensive topic. More research needs to be done to determine if there are different outcomes between groups of people whose medical costs were paid for with bundled payment methods or FFS. As well, more conclusive research needs to be done on how provider behavior is influenced by cost-containment strategies. Knowing this type of information could aid our country's quest for more affordable and higher quality health care.

SUMMARY

Cost control is an attempt to decrease the overall flow of money into financing and/or reimbursing health care. There are financing controls, reimbursement controls, and mixed controls.

Financing controls consist of regulatory and competitive strategies to decrease the flow of money into health care. It is thought that by limiting the funding for health care (financing), we will simultaneously limit the spending on health care (reimbursement). Financing controls are thought to be the weaker cost-control strategy, because ultimately these methods do not keep the cost of taxes and/or premiums for health insurance down.

Reimbursement controls include price and utilization controls. Price controls consist of regulation and competitive strategies for cost control, such as government regulation of Medicare or payer-provider negotiations for competitive fee schedules.

Utilization controls consist of bundled payments, cost sharing, utilization management, and supply limits. More focus has been on reimbursement cost-control strategies because they are thought to be more effective.

The effectiveness of these cost-control strategies is not yet understood. Some research suggests that these controls do make a difference in health care costs; however, other research does not show this. More outcomes research needs to be done in this area to study the effects of various cost-control methods on both health care costs and patient outcomes and to clear up the ambiguity and inconsistencies of previous research.

REFERENCES

1. Bodenheimer TS, Grumbach K. *Understanding Health Policy: A Clinical Approach.* Stamford, CT: Appleton and Lange; 1995.
2. Hoffman C, Rice D, Sung HY. Persons with chronic conditions: their prevalence and costs. *JAMA.* 1996;276(18):1473-1479.
3. Chronic care needs on the rise. *PT Bulletin.* 1996;11(47):1, 10.
4. Lumsdon K. Working smarter, not harder. *Hospitals & Health Networks.* 1995;26(21):27-31.
5. Alzheimer's treatment costs could bankrupt Medicare, The Health Care News Server. http://www.healthcarenewsserver.com/stories/HCN1998032400008.shtml, 3/25/98.

6. Grumbach K, Bodenheimer TS. Mechanisms for controlling costs. *JAMA.* 1995;273(15):1223-1229.

7. Newhouse JP, Manning WG, Morris CN, et al. Some interim results from a controlled trial of cost sharing in health insurance. *N Engl J Med.* 1981;305(25):1501-1507.

8. Letsch SW, Lazenby HC, Levit KR, Conan DA. National health care expenditures, 1991. *Health Care Financing Review.* 1992;14(2):1-17.

9. Gramm P. Why we need medical savings accounts. *N Engl J Med.* 1994;330(24):1752-1753.

10. Keeler EB, Malkin JD, Goldman DP, Buchanan JL. Can medical savings accounts for the nonelderly reduce health care costs? *JAMA.* 1996;275(21):1666-1671.

11. Stewart DL, Abeln SH. *Documenting Functional Outcomes in Physical Therapy.* St. Louis, MO: Mosby-Year Book, Inc.; 1993.

12. *The Balanced Budget Act: How it Affects Physical Therapy;* American Physical Therapy Association. http://www.apta.org/govt_aff/bbasynop.html, 4/6/98.

13. Relman AS. Assessment and accountability: the third revolution in medical care. *N Engl J Med.* 1988;319(18):1220-1222.

14. Stewart DL, Abeln SH. *Documenting Functional Outcomes in Physical Therapy.* St. Louis, MO: Mosby-Year Book, Inc.; 1993.

15. Siu AL, Sonnenberg FA, Manning WG, et al. Inappropriate use of hospitals in a randomized trial of health care services. *N Engl J Med.* 1986;315:1259-1266.

16. Clifton DW. A shift towards utilization management. *PT-Magazine of Physical Therapy.* 1995;3(6):32-35.

17 Kerr EA, Mittman BS, Hays RD, Siu AL, Leake B, Brook R. Managed care and capitation in California: how do physicians at financial risk control their own utilization? *Ann Intern Med.* 1995;123(7):500-504.

18. Wennberg JE, Gittelsohn A. Small area variations in health care delivery. *Science.* 1973;182:1102-1108.

19. Wennberg JE. The paradox of appropriate care. *JAMA.* 1987;258(18):2568-2569.

20. Every NR, Larson EB, Litwin PE, et al. The association between on-site cardiac catheterization facilities and the use of coronary angiography after acute myocardial infarction. *N Engl J Med.* 1993;329(8):546-551.

21. Kane JT, Gallaher AJ, Davis DM, Cummings V. Diagnostic-related groups: their impact on an inpatient rehabilitation program. *Arch Phys Med Rehab.* 1987;68:833-836.

22. Goldman DP, Hosek SD, Dixon LS, Sloss EM. The effects of benefit design and managed care on health care costs. *Journal of Health Economics.* 1995;14:401-418.

23. Hillman AL, Pauly MV, Kerstein J. How do financial incentives affect physicians' clinical decisions and the financial performance of health maintenance organizations? *N Engl J Med.* 1989;321(2):86-92.

24. Buchanan JL, Leibowitz A, Keesey J. Medicaid health maintenance organizations: can they reduce program spending? *Medical Care.* 1996;34(3):249-263.

TEST YOUR SKILLS

Cost-containment strategies (intrasystem)

1. Group patients for treatment
2. Bedside treatments or on-floor treatments
3. Delegate treatment to a multi-skilled worker
4. Chart by exception
5. Family education to provide some aspects of treatment
6. Critical pathways to eliminate routine orders and planning
7. Team conferences/transdisciplinary involvement
8. Educational classes prior to discharge
9. Prewritten educational materials
10. Decrease frequency of physical therapy treatments
11. Decrease total duration of physical therapy treatments
12. Decrease length of individual physical therapy sessions
13. Checklists and inventories in place of social histories and home evaluations
14. Electronic medical records
15. Preventative measures
16. Utilize less labor-intensive treatments

Discuss how each of the above cost-containment strategies could be used in each of the following settings. You may add to the list of strategies above with your own creative innovations. Then discuss the details of implementing them.

1. Acute hospital
2. Skilled nursing facility or sub-acute facility
3. Home health care
4. Outpatient facility

CHECK YOUR RESPONSES

Acute hospital
The following are possible strategies to deal with cost containment at the acute hospital level: #2, 3, 4, 6, 7, 9, 12, 13, 14, 15, 16.

Skilled nursing facility (SNF) and sub-acute facility
The following are possible strategies to deal with cost containment at the SNF level: #1, 3, 5, 6, 7, 8, 10, 11, 12, 13, 14, 15, 16.

Home health care
The following are possible strategies to deal with cost containment at the home health level of care: #5, 6, 7, 9, 10, 11, 12, 13, 14, 15, 16.

Outpatient facility
The following are possible strategies to deal with cost containment in an outpatient clinic: #1, 3, 5, 6, 8, 9, 10, 11, 12, 13, 14, 15, 16.

Implementing cost-containment strategies
Group patients for treatments—This strategy works well for groups of patients of similar functional levels or diagnoses. For example, chair exercises can be done as a group while adequate supervision is provided.

Bedside treatments or on-floor treatments—Physical therapists can save time by treating patients in their rooms, by avoiding the need to transport the patients from their rooms to a distant clinic. This also takes less of the patient's time and energy. Toilet transfers, balance training while dressing, and learning bed and chair transfers become more meaningful to the patient.

Delegate treatment to a multi-skilled worker—Many tasks performed in physical therapy can be performed by a multi-skilled worker with proper training and supervision. Treatment activities, such as modalities, routine therapeutic exercise, dressing, patient transport, answering phones, and equipment maintenance are just a few examples of what can be delegated, freeing up the physical therapist to perform more skilled interventions with patients.

Chart by exception—When using critical pathways, chart only the unexpected. Save time by limiting your comments to only pertinent information that has caused the patient to deviate from the expected plan of treatment.

Family education to provide some aspects of treatment—Teach the family how to assist the patient with the home exercise program. This frees up your treatment time so that you can focus on other important matters that require your skilled intervention as a physical therapist.

Critical pathways to eliminate routine orders and planning—Common medical and surgical diagnoses are appropriate for the development of critical pathways. In addition, some physicians have specific protocols for specific cases or procedures. Take advantage of what you know about these protocols to create a critical pathway that coordinates the services of many disciplines. This often eliminates waiting time for referrals and treatment planning.

Team conferences/transdisciplinary involvement—Weekly meetings with other involved team members (ie, physicians, nurses, respiratory therapists, speech pathologists, occupational therapists, physical therapists, discharge planners, pharmacist, dietician) can enhance decisions and discharge planning for patients.

Educational classes prior to discharge—Offer classes on material that all patients need to know. For example, develop a low back pain education class that teaches proper body mechanics and progresses patients through various levels of exercises.

Prewritten educational materials—Providing written materials during the pre-operative phase for therapy helps patients anticipate what is expected. Pre-written home exercise programs are a big time saver for the busy therapist. Basic exercise routines for various diagnoses and levels of function are useful to have on hand. Many programs are also computerized for easy customization.

Decrease frequency of physical therapy treatments—Teach the patients how to perform their own self-care and home exercise programs. Rely on the patients to follow through with this and progress, while monitoring their treatment program during therapy visits. Consider alternatives to daily or three times weekly treatment as the patient shows progress. Build this into the patient's expectations as well. This also helps to shift the responsibility to the patient.

Decrease total duration of physical therapy treatments—Limit the patient's length of stay in the hospital or duration of treatment by earlier discharge. Instead of treating patients for longer durations, give them the tools they need to progress to an acceptable level of recovery (ie, self-care techniques, pain management, home exercise program, proper posture/body mechanics, preventative care). Schedule follow-up re-evaluation at specific intervals to monitor progress.

Decrease length of individual physical therapy sessions—Limit or decrease individual physical therapy sessions to 30 minutes of the patient's time in the clinic. This can be achieved by limiting the number of modalities or procedures done with each patient. Try to schedule the patient with others who need similar treatment or information.

Checklists and inventories in place of social histories and home evaluations—This can save a clinician much time and effort if a comprehensive checklist is used when evaluating a home setting or inquiring about a social history. In addition, a capable family member may be able to assist greatly with this process.

Electronic medical records—Many of these computerized systems are now available. A computerized documentation system can be set up to track patient characteristics, outcomes, time used, and associated costs, in addition to facilitating billing and record-keeping functions.

Preventative measures—Incorporate "wellness," health promotion, or injury prevention programs into patient education efforts. This will help to prevent future episodes of illness of injury related to a patient's current problem. Give patients the information they need to maximize function and avoid re-injury.

Use less labor-intensive treatments—Use procedures and exercises that require less one-on-one attention. Consider other means of service delivery that maximize physical therapist time, such as interactive computerized patient education programs or videos, preset treatment targets, and group treatment sessions.

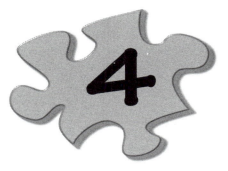

REFERRAL AND ACCESS TO PHYSICAL THERAPY SERVICES

Tod Steffenilla, MPT

Access, our ability to obtain health services when needed, is a hot topic on today's health care agenda.[1] This chapter discusses the factors that influence access in today's health care environment, specifically how patients get to physical therapy, the relationship of access and reimbursement, and barriers that may inhibit the patient from accessing physical therapy services.

Although it varies from state to state, there are essentially two ways the patient can access physical therapy services. One way is with a referral from another health care practitioner such as a physician, osteopath, dentist, podiatrist, or psychologist.[2] A second way to access physical therapy services is with the utilization of direct access to physical therapy. The second method, direct access, varies greatly in legality and practicality from state to state. First, we will look at the historically dominant form of accessing physical therapy services: referral from the health care practitioner.

ACCESSING PHYSICAL THERAPY SERVICES WITH PHYSICIAN REFERRAL

Physician referral accounts for the largest portion of physical therapy referrals from health care practitioners. Physicians refer patients to physical therapists for many different reasons.

Jane Malleolus suffered a grade II ankle sprain during a soccer game. She was taken to her independent practice association-model health maintenance organization's primary care physician later that same day. After a brief examination and instruction to use rest, ice, compression, and elevation, the physician gave her a referral to see a physical therapist.

John Valsalva scheduled and underwent a coronary artery bypass graft procedure at a private hospital that was on the provider list of his preferred provider organization. Soon after his surgery, John was referred to one of the facility's physical therapists by his thoracic surgeon.

The above two examples demonstrate how patients access physical therapy after either an acute trauma or a scheduled surgery. Patients are also referred when they are in need of long-term care, such as home health or nursing home care, or if it is indicated as part of a critical pathway.

Who Pays for Services After the Referral?

Health care insurance coverage determines access to physical therapy services. Payer policies determine the availability of health care services to most of the population.

The principal source of health insurance in the United States is employment-based private insurance, as is demonstrated in Table 4.1. Although the following figures incorporate all US residents, it is important to note that the 36 million Americans living below the poverty line reflect a radically different picture. Twice as many (31%) lack insurance coverage, and twice as many (55%) are covered by government programs, primarily Medicaid (45%).[3]

Benefits and group policies

The group or individual policies and their benefits vary from group to group and from individual to individual. For group health policies, insurance contract negotiations typically begin with a standard contract. The insurer already has constructed a package of health insurance benefits for the standard contract. During negotiations, the employer or its representative (the group administrator) might elect to add or delete certain benefits or to change certain benefit levels. In negotiating group health benefits, it is the employer who really controls the benefits.[4]

Some of the forms of managed care programs are the preferred provider organization (PPO), health maintenance organization (HMO) group or staff model, and independent practice association (IPA) HMOs. There are numerous programs across the United States, and they all differ in services available and

TABLE 4.1

HEALTH INSURANCE COVERAGE STATUS AND TYPE: 1996

	(Numbers in millions)	Percentage
Total covered	225	84.4
Private	187	70.2
• Employment-based	163	61.2
• Government	69	25.9
• Medicare	35	13.2
• Medicaid	31	11.8
• Military	8	3.3
Not covered	42	15.6
Total population	267	100

Source: Current Population Survey. *Washington, DC: US Census Bureau; March 1997*

reimbursement methods. Most notable to the physical therapist is the Kaiser Permanente staff model HMO in which, theoretically, patients should have unlimited access to physical therapy services because of the patient's prepaid status. The treatment that each patient receives is at the discretion of the physical therapist; there really are no reimbursement issues other than maintaining cost effectiveness.[5] This is not the case with federally funded public insurance programs.

Joe Stockboy has been receiving physical therapy for six visits since he injured his arm playing basketball 1 month ago. He has been covered through his employer-based group health insurance, but his allocated visits have been used. You feel Joe would benefit from three more visits. Do you call the insurer or the employer for additional benefits?

Benefits and government-funded programs

Medicare and Medicaid are the two primary sources of government-funded programs. Under Medicare Part A, after the deductible is paid, physical therapy services are covered 100% for the first 60 days of hospitalization. Then, graduated payments are made until the 91st day when no more benefits can be received. One hundred percent coverage is also provided for physical therapy home health care under Part A. Skilled nursing physical therapy care is covered 100% for the first 20 days, and then the patient pays a portion of the fees under Part B until the 101st day. Hospice care is covered 100% for most services, and long-term care has some coverage but is very limited.[1]

Medicare Part B will cover 80% of allowed medical expenses once the annual deductible has been paid but will limit the dollar amount per year for outpatient and long-term care physical therapy services.[6] With the implementation of the 1997 Balanced Budget Amendment, access to physical therapy services will likely change with changes in coverage.

Medicaid is a federal- and state-run program that is designed to provide medical coverage to people who meet certain income limits. Medicaid covers hospitalization, nursing home, and home health (limited), and states can add to or limit any or all of these services.[1] Medicaid coverage for physical therapy services has traditionally been quite low, but varies widely by state. Some states are now channeling their funds for Medicaid benefits instead to HMOs in exchange for their management of these patients. This may improve access to services for the poor, as historically, health care providers have turned these patients away due to difficulty meeting their costs with the minimal reimbursement offered by Medicaid programs in many states.

More than 31 million people are covered by Medicaid; however, almost 42 million lack health insurance coverage.[3] How do the uninsured access physical therapy services?

Workers' compensation programs

A second form of state-regulated insurance programs are workers' compensation programs. The programs themselves may not be state run, but the fee scheduling of the provider is typically set by government agencies that are responsible for "overseeing" the programs. Several methods of coverage and reimbursement are currently being tested. Some of the current trends are 24-hour coverage, resource-based relative value system (RBRVS)-based fee schedules, and cascading coverage. Each of these methods may affect patient access to physical therapy services in its own way, either directly or indirectly.

Twenty-four-hour coverage is when the employee's health care plan covers him or her on and off the job "24 hours." The advantages of this plan include no change in payments made by the employer and no change in benefits to employees whether using their employment-based group health insurance coverage or workers' compensation insurance. Additionally, there would be no reason for the injured party to report that the injury took place at work when in fact it did not.[7] This would then lead to a decrease in workers' compensation fraud and allow the therapist to obtain a more accurate history from the patient as to the mode of injury. More accurate information may lead to a more comprehensive evaluation and better management of the patient's injury.

A second trend is to reimburse the workers' compensation provider using the *RBRVS-based fee schedule*s.[7] The RBRVS is used in the reimbursement of

Medicare patients. One author states, "...the health care needs of a 24-year-old construction worker with an injury can be expected to differ significantly from those of a 72-year-old retiree with a chronic condition."[7] Taking notice of this difference in patient population, some states have adjusted the payment schedule accordingly by adding a certain percentage on top of the fee schedule. Even with the added percentage, reimbursement for these workers' compensation patients will still be lower to the physical therapist accepting these patients.

A third trend is the *cascading payment*. This works to set a limit on the fee schedule for workers' compensation. The cascade operates on the premise that only the initial procedure will be reimbursed at 100% of a predetermined fee schedule. The second procedure is reimbursed at 75%, the third procedure at 50%, and any others at 25% of their scheduled value. This method was brought about by insurers that had clients undergoing multiple surgical procedures, and they felt they should only pay in full for the primary procedure because the patient was already prepared for additional procedures.[7] Currently, not enough data are gathered to tell if this is an effective way to pay for physical therapy services rendered in a workers' compensation claim because of the time-based nature of physical therapy billing codes.

ACCESSING PHYSICAL THERAPY SERVICES USING DIRECT ACCESS

Pure direct access is defined by Anderson as "the ability to treat clients needing physical therapy without forced outside intervention."[8] Even in the states that do allow evaluation and treatment without a referral, as opposed to the states that only allow evaluation, there are often stipulations that inhibit "pure" direct access. With varying restrictions to direct access in each state, we will use the term *direct access* for all cases in which the patient accesses physical therapy services without the referral of another health care practitioner.

The legality of direct access varies from state to state. Forty-five states allow physical therapy evaluation only without a referral, and 31 states allow evaluation and treatment without referral. See Table 4.2 to check your state.

Accessing physical therapy as a primary care choice for patients may be the key to receiving physical therapy services in a timely manner, which historically has been a problem. One study reports that patients themselves often delay seeking health care. Patients cite cost and inconvenience in obtaining a referral for physical therapy as the reason for their delay in seeking treatment

TABLE 4.2

DIRECT ACCESS PER PT PRACTICE ACTS (BY STATE)

States that permit PT evaluation without physician referral	States that permit PT treatment without physician referral
Alaska	Alaska
Arizona	Arizona
Arkansas	Arkansas
California	California
Colorado	Colorado
Connecticut	Delaware
Delaware	Florida
Florida	Idaho
Georgia	Illinois
Hawaii	Iowa
Idaho	Kentucky
Illinois	Maine
Iowa	Maryland
Kansas	Massachusetts
Kentucky	Minnesota
Louisiana	Montana
Maine	Nebraska
Maryland	Nevada
Massachusetts	New Hampshire
Michigan	New Mexico
Minnesota	North Carolina
Mississippi	North Dakota
Montana	Oregon
Nebraska	Rhode Island
Nevada	South Dakota
New Hampshire	Texas
New Jersey	Utah
New Mexico	Vermont
New York	Washington
North Carolina	West Virginia
North Dakota	Wisconsin
Oklahoma	*Total: 31*
Oregon	
Pennsylvania	
Rhode Island	**States without direct access**
South Dakota	Alabama
Tennessee	Indiana
Texas	Missouri
Utah	Ohio
Vermont	South Carolina
South Carolina	*Total: 5*
Washington	
Washington DC	
West Virginia	
Wisconsin	
Wyoming	
Total: 45	

Reprinted from Physical Therapy Without Referral. *Alexandria, Va: American Physical Therapy Association; 1997, with permission from the American Physical Therapy Association.*

or for choosing an alternate, less traditional form of treatment. With this delay in appropriate medical care, they risk exacerbating their physical disability and damaging their health.[2]

Primary Care

The reality of the physical therapist becoming the primary entry point for patients, or part of a primary care team, is already in place in some states, and steps are being taken in others to make it possible and practical. Two examples are the University of North Carolina (UNC) and the Northern California Kaiser Permanente system.

UNC has a model for a primary care team approach. The team consists of a physical therapist, a geriatrician, a nurse practitioner, a social worker, a pharmacist, and a geriopsychiatrist.[9] This primary care team is mobile and visits those rural areas in which the residents do not have easy access to physical therapy or health care in general.

In the Northern California Kaiser Permanente system, a training program has been proposed for physical therapists to act as primary care providers for patients with musculoskeletal disorders. The program has been implemented in several pilot clinics. This is a big step for patient access to physical therapy services and, as stated by Carol Jo Tichenor, "is potentially the most important change in the role of physical therapists in the history of our organization."[10]

The proposed training for entry into a primary care role consists of educational courses in medical differential diagnosis, acute management of musculoskeletal conditions, radiology, pharmacology, laboratory technology, team building, and communication skills. This educational experience may be enhanced through the mentoring program in Orthopedic Manual Therapy at Kaiser Hayward (Calif).

The therapist trained in the adult primary care (APC) role would work in outpatient medical clinics. The APC team would consist of physicians, nurse practitioners, a behavioral medicine specialist, a physical therapist, and a health education specialist. Each team member has the responsibility to refer patients appropriately within the team and to outside specialists when indicated. In some of the pilot clinics that have already been implemented, patients are referred to physical therapy after a "quick screen" by a physician, while in other clinics the patient is screened over the phone to check for musculoskeletal problems prior to accessing a primary care therapist.

If the primary care therapist determines the patient will need ongoing physical therapy, he or she will be referred directly to the physical therapy department. Ultimately, the goal would be referral of patients with musculoskeletal disorders directly to a physical therapist as a "first contact provider."[10]

With physical therapists as integral members of an APC, patients are able to access the most skilled provider for their physical therapy problems upon entry into the health care system and can become involved in their rehabilitation without the delay of seeking a referral from another practitioner.[10] In the above two examples, we can see that physical therapist roles in primary care are under development, and exciting new changes are already taking place. This new service delivery model for physical therapy should have benefits to both the patient and the profession.

Military Model

The military model of physical therapy is already designed in such a way that patients are sure to obtain the proper intervention in an appropriate timeframe. Physical therapists in the military are not bound by state laws and regulations as long as they are practicing on a military installation. Military therapists are given "clinical privileges" that enable them to be primary care providers to appropriate patients with neuromusculoskeletal disorders. These clinical privileges are based on experience and education. Some privileges differ from those that civilian therapists can exercise. Military therapists can request radiological studies be carried out and interpreted, and they may prescribe medications, like nonsteroidal anti-inflammatories and non-narcotic muscle relaxants.[11]

The typical patient is screened for vital signs and other pertinent history and then, if appropriate, is seen by a physical therapist. The patient may, in fact, be screened by the physical therapist. The therapist will then perform an evaluation, assess the patient's functional limitations, and assign a diagnosis. The therapist will also delineate an appropriate treatment plan. If the patient's

Joe Lumbardi hurt his low back while mountain biking on his weekend off. Joe's good friend recommended a chiropractor because he knew Joe had no comprehensive health care coverage, and the chiropractor has a special discount for first-time visitors. Joe had a chiropractic evaluation and three follow-up visits. He had relief for about a week; and then for the next 3 months he had a nagging low back problem interfering with his ability to work. Joe changed jobs and eventually received health care benefits that included comprehensive health care. Joe then visited a physician who promptly referred him to physical therapy for evaluation and treatment. Would Joe have possibly benefited from earlier access to physical therapy? Could he have used direct access to a physical therapist?

needs are beyond the scope of the therapist or if the therapist wishes to consult with the physician, the military model of physical therapy ensures immediate access to other health care members.[11] The military has been using this model for some 18 years; and thus far, it has proven to be efficient and cost effective for them and may well be the model of the future for civilian physical therapy as well.

Who Pays for Services Using Direct Access?

Although most states permit some form of direct access to physical therapy services, one of the main barriers to its utilization is the lack of reimbursement from third-party payers. One reason that insurers have shown a lack of willingness to reimburse for services rendered without a physician referral is their fear of an increase in malpractice claims. This fear has proven to be unfounded as evidenced by a letter written by Maginnis and Associates, a large provider of professional liability insurance, in consultation with the Washington State Physical Therapy Association in which "no change in claim frequency or severity" has been noted (written communication, 1990).

Comparing the current listing (Table 4.3) with a listing published a few years ago, it appears that the trend is for more third-party payers to accept and pay for direct access to physical therapy services. The lack of reimbursement across the board among insurers is what causes many to believe that it is not practical to practice strictly through direct access.

The thought of all patients coming to physical therapists exclusively without referral is not realistic, nor is it the intent of direct access. Physical therapists will continue to work with physicians and other health care practitioners through referrals. Direct access will not stop this process. It will only serve to let physicians treat patients who require their medical expertise without the added load of patients who are coming to them simply for a referral to physical therapy.

Aside from insurer hesitancy to reimburse, opposition to direct access comes in a large part from three groups: chiropractors, physicians, and other physical therapists. A Texas American Physical Therapy Association fact sheet presented the following (Page 77):

TABLE 4.3

INSURERS PAYING FOR PT EVALUATION WITHOUT PHYSICIAN REFERRAL

Evaluation	Treatment
Aetna	CT, IL, IA, KY, MD, NY, NC, TX*, VT
Blue Cross	AR, CA (Shield)*, CO, ID, IL, KY*, MD, MA, MN, MT, NC, SD, VT, WA (Eastern WA-BS*)
Cigna	AR, CN, IA, LA, NC, TX
Equitable	IL, IA, MD, MN, NY, NC, TX
John Hancock	IL, MD
Metropolitan	CO, CN, KY*, MD, NY
Mutual of Omaha	KY*, MT
New York Life	MD, MT
Prudential	CT, KY*, MD*, MT, NY
State Farm	KY
Travelers	IL, KY*, MD, NY, VT, MT
Great West	MD*
Susquehanna	MD*
SAMBA	MD*
First Choice Health Network	WA*
Aetna	IA, KY, NC, VT
Blue Cross	AR, CA (Shield)*, CO, ID, IA, KY, MD, MA, MT, NC, SD, VT, WA (Eastern WA-BS*)
Cigna	AR, IA, NC
Equitable	IA, IL, MD, MN, NC
John Hancock	MD
Metropolitan	CO, KY
Mutual of Omaha	MT
New York Life	MD, MT
Prudential	KY, MD, MT
State Farm	KY
Travelers	MD, MT, VT
Transamerica	MD, MT, VT
Virginia Mason Health Plan	WA*
First Choice Health Network	WA*

*Under certain conditions/coverages

Reprinted from Physical Therapy without Referral. *Alexandria, Va: American Physical Therapy Association; 1997, with permission from the American Physical Therapy Association.*

- *Chiropractors—They have worked hard to build their current image, which was given a boost when chiropractic care was approved for insurance coverage. They do not want the competition of physical therapists since the consumer would have the alternative to go to a physical therapist under direct access.*
- *Physicians—Many physicians fear that with direct access to physical therapy, many patients or the management of their treatment will be lost, as it has with chiropractic services. In reality, the experience that direct access states has revealed that the medical loop is very much intact, but in a more efficient manner.*
- *Other physical therapists—As in all professions, there are some who disagree with a nationwide trend. A small minority of physical therapists are not in favor of direct access. With direct access passed in Texas, they will not be required to accept patients without a referral; they too will have a choice.[12]*

BARRIERS IN ACCESSING PHYSICAL THERAPY SERVICES

Some of the barriers that patients encounter in accessing physical therapy services are lack of insurance coverage, insurance limits to frequency, duration or total costs of services, location, and gatekeepers. Additional barriers include lack of knowledge in the public at large and other health care workers as to the capabilities of physical therapy and availability of physical therapy services. How many of these barriers have you personally witnessed? First, we will look at lack of insurance coverage.

Lack of health care insurance coverage or payer-imposed limits to the frequency, duration, or total costs of physical therapy are two of the more common barriers that limit patient access to physical therapy services. Almost 16% of the American population is without health care coverage.[3] The inability of this group to access the type of care that they require is one reason that community outreach programs and volunteer hours at free screening clinics are so important to the health of American citizens. With the need for health care cost containment, many services are being restricted or removed from health care plans. Physical therapy is not exempt from this budget axe.

"Some payers want therapists to see the patient on postoperative day 1... and then see the patient on the day of discharge... Others are making a unilateral decision that physical therapy is 'not necessary' or can be provided by non-physical therapy staff."[13] These are primary reasons that physical therapists must be pro-active in defining their professional role and their patients' need for professional skill-level services.

Location has long been a barrier to physical therapy services. Many patients in rural communities may lack access to physical therapy services.

One sound alternative to this problem is that of mobile primary care teams (like that at the University of North Carolina) who travel to rural sites to provide needed care.

Many times, although physical therapy services are covered, the patient sometimes finds a barrier at the level of the primary care physician or "gatekeeper." This may have an origin in one of two perspectives:

1. The third-party payer or physician's perspective on cost containment: Remember that in many capitated health plans, the IPA receives a set amount of money and any referrals that member physicians make come from the IPA budget.
2. A lack of understanding from the referring health care practitioner or the patients themselves as to the need for, efficacy of, or scope of services that physical therapists offer. Good interprofessional communication and public education will help to educate professionals and patients.

> *Susan Cheeks came to the outpatient physical therapy clinic at her group model HMO 1 week after the onset of Bell's palsy. When asked why she had not been referred earlier, she said that her physician at the HMO said there was nothing physical therapy could do to help her. After 1 week, she was scared and frustrated about her condition. Susan went outside of her HMO to seek medical advice. A nurse practitioner sent her back to her HMO physician and advised that she may benefit from physical therapy services. You, as the physical therapist, treat her for 2 weeks and see marked improvement of her physical and mental health since the onset of treatment. Should the physician know that there are treatment options for this condition?*

SUMMARY

This chapter was designed to show how patients access physical therapy services, the relationship of reimbursement to access, and some of the barriers to accessing physical therapy services. It is beyond the scope of this chapter to explore every aspect involved with access issues. However, physical therapists need to be aware of barriers preventing access to services in their communities and educate payers, potential referral sources, and the public.

Being active in legislative processes concerning direct access and participating in free community screening clinics are two ways in which physical therapists may, themselves, help to increase patient access to physical therapy services. In today's health care environment, physical therapists are challenged to be innovative to ensure access to the services of physical therapy that can help so many people.

REFERENCES

1. Bodenheimer TS, Grumbach K. *Understanding Health Policy—A Clinical Approach.* Stamford, Conn: Appleton and Lange; 1995.
2. Durant T, Lord L, Domholdt E. Outpatient views on direct access to physical therapy in Indiana. *Phys Ther.* 1989;69(10):850-857.
3. U.S. Census Bureau, *March 1997 Current Population Survey.* http://www.census.gov/hhes/hlthins/cover96.html, 6/26/98.
4. Lanes D. How the claims process works. *PT-Magazine of Physical Therapy.* 1996;4(5):30-32.
5. Thornbury, Sharon. Director of physical therapy services, Kaiser Permanente Medical Center, Personal interview. Fresno, Calif. April 15, 1997.
6. Davolt S. Tender loving Medicare. *PT-Magazine of Physical Therapy.* 1996;4(12):50-52.
7. Lansey D. Trends in Workers' Compensation reimbursement. *PT-Magazine of Physical Therapy.* 1996;4(10):20-22.
8. Anderson L. 1989 American Physical Therapy Association Board of Directors and Officers elections. *Progress Report of the American Physical Therapy Association.* 1989;18(3):19.
9. Monahan B. Autonomy, access, and choice: New models for primary care. *PT-Magazine of Physical Therapy.* 1996;4(9):54-58.
10. Tichenor CJ. Kaiser Permanente moves forward with physical therapists in primary care. *California Chapter American Physical Therapy Association Newsletter.* 1997;30(11):1.
11. Spillane D. Step into the "military model" of PT practice. *California Chapter American Physical Therapy Association Newsletter.* 1997;30(2): 1.
12. *Texas Physical Therapy Association Fact Sheet. Topic: Proponents and opponents to direct access.* Alexandria, Va: American Physical Therapy Association; 1997.
13. Reynolds JP. LOS: SOS? You could say that managed care ultimately is about one thing: discharge planning. *PT-Magazine of Physical Therapy.* 1996;4(2):38-46.
14. *Physical therapy without referral: Direct Access (packet),* 1997. Government Affairs Department, Alexandria, Va: American Physical Therapy Association, 1997.

TEST YOUR SKILLS

1. Explain two ways in which a patient can access physical therapy services.
2. Name five different types of health care practitioners who refer patients to physical therapy.
3. Name the principal source of health insurance coverage in the United States.
4. Name three forms of managed care coverage through which a potential patient could access physical therapy services.
5. Define the term *pure direct access*.
6. How many states have legalized direct access to physical therapy for evaluation only? For evaluation and treatment?
7. Is direct access legal in your state? In what capacity?
8. How many insurers will reimburse for services rendered using direct access? Are there any in your state?
9. What are some benefits of direct access for the patient? For the physical therapist?
10. What are some barriers to accessing physical therapy services?

CHECK YOUR RESPONSES

1. Two ways for a patient to access physical therapy services:
    (1) With a referral from a health care practitioner
    (2) Through direct access
2. Five types of health care practitioners who refer a patient for physical therapy services are
    (1) Physician
    (2) Osteopath
    (3) Dentist
    (4) Podiatrist
    (5) Psychologist
    Additional practitioners may be able to refer patients in many community and clinical settings.
3. The principal source of health care coverage in the United States is employment-based private insurance.
4. Three managed care programs through which a potential patient could access physical therapy services are PPOs, group or staff model HMOs, or IPAs.
5. *Pure direct access* is described in the literature as "the ability to treat clients needing physical therapy without forced outside intervention."[8]
6. Forty-five states have legalized direct access to physical therapy for evaluation only, while 31 states allow evaluation and treatment (see Table 4.2).
7. See Table 4.2 to find the status of direct access in your state.
8. There are currently 17 insurers that reimburse for the variations of direct access. See Table 4.3 for a complete listing of those available in your state.
9. Some possible benefits of direct access for the patient are decreases in cost, inconvenience, and the likelihood of exacerbation of symptoms prior to receiving the appropriate care. Possible benefits to the therapist are increased autonomy of practice and the opportunity to treat a patient in the beginning stages of an injury, prior to the condition becoming chronic, increasing the likelihood of successfully treating the patient.
10. Some potential barriers to physical therapy services are lack of insurance, insurance limits to frequency, duration, or annual costs of physical therapy, rural or under-served locations, lack of referrals from gatekeepers, and the lack of knowledge of other health care practitioners and the public at large as to the role and scope of physical therapy.

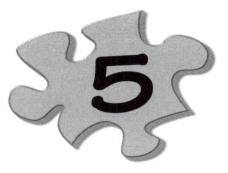

TRENDS & STRATEGIES FOR PHYSICAL THERAPY PRACTICE IN ACUTE CARE

Sonya Yokes, MPT

Health care in acute hospitals has markedly changed in the past two decades. This chapter discusses the continuing evolution of the acute care setting and how these changes have affected the practice of physical therapy. By understanding the nature of these changes and the factors influencing the focus of practice, physical therapists can develop effective patient management strategies.

Jeanette Stiles recently graduated with a master's degree in physical therapy. She attended a state physical therapy conference and talked with personnel from a large acute hospital who had booths for therapist recruitment at the conference. She wants to work in an acute teaching hospital because of the wide variety of patients, the pace, and the excitement of working with the latest technology and advances in medicine. She is elated when she receives a telephone call asking her to come in for an interview.

PHYSICAL THERAPY AND ACUTE CARE

More physical therapists work in acute care hospitals than in any other practice setting. New graduate physical therapists often seek acute care practice positions to gain experience and exposure to a variety of patient diagnoses.[1] These therapists often leave the setting after several years, going on to opportunities in other areas of practice. High turnover rates and staffing shortages are widespread in many acute hospitals and complicate some of the patient management challenges that acute care therapists face.[1] Let's look first at some of the factors that influence practice in this setting.

Co-morbidity

The face of acute care continues to change. The patient population is older and much sicker than ever before.[1] Modern medical technology provides the tools to keep people alive longer, and with this added longevity comes co-morbidity. As medicine controls one illness, it allows time for another illness to develop.

Co-morbidity is the presence of multiple diagnoses requiring management. Physical therapists see many patients with two or more diagnoses. A therapist may be treating a patient after an open reduction internal fixation of a hip fracture, but this patient may also have chronic obstructive pulmonary disease, congestive heart failure, rheumatoid arthritis, and osteoporosis. The therapist must now consider all of these conditions, the effects of medications, and related contraindications and precautions while treating the patient. This also means that the therapist must have knowledge of the pathology and pharmacology associated with the patient's diagnoses as well as in-depth knowledge of the musculoskeletal system.[2,3]

Decreased Length of Stay

Ralph Jorgenson, a 68-year-old insulin-dependent diabetic, was admitted on Sunday afternoon, unconscious, after collapsing at his granddaughter's soccer match. He was diagnosed with heat exhaustion. He was monitored overnight and hydrated with intravenous fluids. On Monday morning, he was conscious but quite groggy. His doctor came to check on him and informed Mr. Jorgenson that his stay was no longer medically necessary and that he must call his wife to arrange for transportation home.

Chapters 2 and 3 discussed the influence of the Medicare prospective payment system in shortening acute care length of stay (LOS) by providing a financial incentive for early discharge. The hospital stays of most patients have been cut by two thirds since the introduction of this system in the mid 1980s. The average length of stay 15 years ago was 14 to 16 days. Five years ago, the average length of stay was 6 to 8 days.[4] Today, the average length of stay for a patient in an acute care setting in the United States is 5 days.[5,6]

This means several things: First, patients are going home sicker. Second, physical therapy services must be initiated sooner.[2] Therefore, physical therapists are seeing patients who are more critically ill than before. Third, it has been necessary to change the physical therapy goals from achieving full independence to achieving assisted mobility sufficient to go home or to another level of care. Lastly, patients are frequently *re-admitted* to the hospital with additional complications, having failed to reach their previous functional level. These patients may fall into a downward spiral, losing function and developing further complications requiring multiple re-admissions.

The above trends require physical therapists to be especially skilled in the management of complex and challenging patients. Planning for discharge and prevention of future problems has become a focus of physical therapy care, in addition to management of the patient's immediate needs. Communication with other providers is critical to ensure that patient needs are met and that continuity of care is maximized.

Winifred Duncan has lived alone since the death of her husband 5 years ago. She has become increasingly frail and has fallen more and more often in the past few years. She is afraid to leave her apartment because the neighborhood is too dangerous. Last week, she stood on a piano bench to clean her overhead light fixture. She lost her balance and fell to the floor, sustaining a compression fracture of the thoracic spine, several rib fractures, and a right wrist fracture. She has a daughter who lives 600 miles away and no other relatives.

Discharge Planning

Due to decreased LOS, physical therapists must make recommendations about discharge from the moment of first contact with the patient. Therapists play a large part in deciding discharge destination, whether it is to a skilled nursing facility, rehabilitation facility, or home.

To make an informed discharge decision and to plan treatment that will prepare the patient for the next level of care, therapists need to solicit the following information from patients and their families:
1. The patient's prior level of function
2. Home environment (bathroom, stairs, and other barriers)
3. Social support and physical assistance available at home
4. Assistive devices available or in place at home
5. The patient's insurance coverage and payment options for various levels of care

Once this information is gathered, therapists must work with the family and patient to determine patient goals, estimate the time needed to reach these goals, and determine what level of care will best address the needs of the patient.

Prior level of function and availability of social support are likely to play a large part in this decision. A patient with little social support who was previously ambulatory only in his or her home may need considerable intervention at a skilled nursing facility before returning home. In contrast, other patients and families may be able to manage quite well with home health care on immediate discharge.

PRIORITIZING TREATMENT ACTIVITIES

Therapists need to tailor their treatments to accomplish the immediate goals required to move patients to the next level of care and, at the same time, keep in mind the patients' long-term goals of returning to their prior level of function. Given the limited time available and the multiple concerns that often exist, the physical therapist must prioritize treatment activities.

For example, if the patient will be discharged home and has four steps to get into the house, the patient will need to accomplish this goal prior to discharge from the hospital. If this same patient, however, will be going to a rehabilitation unit, the issue of stairs is no longer the focus of treatment. Chapters 8 and 9 may be helpful in managing some of these common practice issues.

PATIENT EDUCATION

Decreased LOS also means that the acute care therapist may not have time to address all patient concerns in an individualized manner. This requires an approach that emphasizes patient education and transfers some responsibility to the patient and family.

There are many effective patient education strategies. First, it is important to involve the patient and family members during treatment. Family members and other caregivers may be the most important link to ensure the patient's well-being after discharge. Therefore, it is important to include them in any patient education strategy.

During a treatment session, therapists can verbally give the patient and his or her family and caregivers information about the patient's condition, what to expect, and what actions need to be independently performed to assist in the healing process. To assist in follow-through, therapists may provide written materials or videos that outline home exercises to be performed, including instructions on how to do the exercises, frequency, repetitions, and duration of each exercise. In addition, an example of a reasonable and safe rate of progression can be described.

The educational process can often begin before admission. Preoperative classes can be held for patients being admitted for elective surgery. These classes can include information about the procedure, what to expect, and actions that the patient can take to make recovery smoother. This prepares the patient for activities that will be necessary to regain function after surgery. It also readies the patient for physical therapy treatment and decreases the amount of time needed for the physical therapist to perform educational instruction.

HOSPITAL RESTRUCTURING & PATIENT-FOCUSED CARE

As the impact of prospective payment systems became more apparent in the 1980s, acute hospitals faced tremendous financial pressures, shortages of staff with appropriate skills, and an increase in competition as well as changing expectations of health care consumers. Hospitals were forced to restructure to contain costs and provide a more consumer-friendly service to increase patient satisfaction.

Large-scale acute hospital restructuring has had a significant influence on physical therapy practice in acute care settings. The initial push for restructuring came from reorganization by hospital management with an increased orientation of the health care system toward those who used the services.

Excessive hierarchies, centralization of services in departments, complex admissions, and diagnostic and treatment processes were not only costly but provided a circuitous and often frustrating journey for the patient to navigate. Improving the patient's experience became the focus of acute hospital reorganization.

Patient-focused care evolved in the early 1990s. This approach was aimed at providing more personalized patient care, improving the continuity of care for patients, facilitating collaborative relationships among health care professionals and caregivers, and centering care around patient needs, rather than hospital departments.

The following are common characteristics of patient-focused care:[3]
- Grouping of patients with similar diagnoses and resource needs
- Decentralization of ancillary services
- Cross-training of employees to produce multi-skilled workers
- Transdisciplinary team approach
- Critical pathways or care paths
- Charting by exception

Let's look below at how each of these elements influences physical therapy care.

Grouping Patients

Grouping of patients with similar diagnoses can be of great benefit to a physical therapist. Having all of the orthopedic patients in one area equates into less travel time for the therapist.

Decentralization

Decentralization is a way to save time and increase continuity of care. Dispersal of support services allows quick, consistent, and convenient access to needed resources at each care site. Decentralized physical therapy service often means that, instead of the patients coming to the physical therapy department, the physical therapist provides services in a more convenient location for the patient.

Management structure also changes with decentralization. One manager is likely to supervise the performance of a larger, multidisciplinary group of professionals. Instead of reporting to a department director, acute care physical therapists may report to a rehabilitation services manager and/or to the manager of a patient-focused specialized unit of care, such as an acute orthopedics service, an oncology unit, a transplant team, or a neonatal unit.

Multi-skilled Workers

This designation usually refers to nonprofessional support personnel who have been cross-trained to provide a variety of technical services in health care delivery. For example, a worker might provide for routine daily patient care needs supervised by nursing and physical therapy. Titles for these workers vary; some facilities call them *care partners*, *care associates*, and *technical partners*.

The American Physical Therapy Association (APTA) position on multi-skilled personnel supports their use as long as they perform under the supervision of physical therapists and physical therapist assistants and in accordance with state laws and regulations:

The American Physical Therapy Association opposes the concept of the multi-skilled professional practitioner, defined as "a health care practitioner who is cross-trained in area(s) of practice in which the individual is neither educated nor licensed." The APTA opposes cross-training of physical therapists and physical therapist assistants in areas outside the scope of physical therapy practice. The APTA also opposes cross-training of other health care practitioners into physical therapy practice. This position should not be interpreted as expressing opposition to coor-

dination of care involving professional practitioners from different disciplines or dual-credentialing through education and licensure.

The APTA supports the utilization of multi-skilled (cross-trained) support personnel who perform delegated components of physical therapy intervention under the direct supervision of physical therapists and physical therapist assistants in accordance with state laws and regulations. Multi-skilled support personnel refers to individuals with "on-the-job training within applicable state laws and regulations to provide services outside or in addition to the scope of their educational preparation or training." When multi-skilled (cross-trained) personnel perform delegated tasks other than those delegated under the direction of a physical therapist, they should be under the direct supervision of an appropriate licensed health care practitioner.[7]

Transdisciplinary Team

The *transdisciplinary team* approach emphasizes optimal communication and coordination of care between all individuals working with a patient. This benefits the patient, family, and health care providers. Everyone can work toward the same goal with the patient and share information. Teamwork cuts down on duplication of efforts and repetition of history-taking and evaluation procedures for the patient and family. With all involved working toward the same goal, the patient is able to reach the goal faster.

Critical Pathways

Critical pathways are time-saving devices that keep patients moving steadily toward discharge. A critical pathway is a "map" that outlines the types of decisions that need to be made, the timelines for applying that information, and the actions that need to be taken based on a given diagnosis. These preset plans save time by eliminating the need to map out a specific sequence of care for each patient. Moreover, critical pathways also contribute to the continuity of patient care (see Appendix 7).

Charting by Exception

Physical therapists spend a large portion of their time charting patient progress and findings. *Charting by exception* is a strategy that can decrease documentation time by 50%. Charting by exception is a shorthand documentation of normal findings for patient assessment and intervention. Further explanation of findings that deviate from normal receive additional documentation.[3]

STRATEGIES

There are numerous strategies that can be employed by physical therapists to provide effective and efficient care in the acute care setting. You may already be using some of these:

- Use time-management techniques (see Chapter 8).
- Use support personnel (aides and assistants) (see Chapter 9).
- Group treatments (two patients in one room being treated simultaneously). For example, two total knee replacement patients can be instructed in bed exercises at the same time. This saves the therapist time and gives both patients a peer with whom to relate.
- Refer patients to nursing for ambulation and transfers when skilled physical therapy is no longer needed.
- Team conferences (transdisciplinary team approach). Good communication between team members decreases duplication of treatment and helps the team work toward the same goal for the patient.
- Critical pathways. Critical pathways can save time by decreasing duplication of documentation and help to progress patients appropriately through their rehabilitation.
- Chart by exception.
- Pre-printed evaluation and treatment forms, as well as check-off lists, can be used for documentation. They make documentation easier to read and save time.
- Computer scheduling to prevent overlapping of transdisciplinary treatments (occupational therapy, physical therapy, rehabilitational therapy).
- Patient education materials assist patients in taking responsibility for their health care and rehabilitation. They can also be a time-saving device.
- Discharge planning at the time of initial evaluation. A physical therapist should start discharge planning as soon as he or she receives information about the patient. The therapist should immediately begin preparing the patient for the next level of care.

Table 5.1 addresses high priority survival skills and training needs for physical therapists who practice in the acute care setting.

TABLE 5.1

ACUTE CARE PHYSICAL THERAPIST'S SURVIVAL SKILLS

SURVIVAL SKILL 1
Addressing highest-priority patient needs
Training needs:
- Develop methods to focus treatment goals and time on highest-priority patient functional needs.
- Assist with problem recognition and effective planning for discharge.

SURVIVAL SKILL 2
Referring to post-discharge care providers
Training needs:
- Increase familiarity with the post-discharge care network.
- Become oriented with range of available community health services.
- Assist with identifying criteria for various levels of post-discharge care.

SURVIVAL SKILL 3
Interpersonal skills with patients
Training needs:
- Improve ability to recognize and resolve patient/provider goal incongruity problems.
- Develop skills in explaining the role and limitations to patients.
- Assist with strategies to work with difficult or demanding patients.

SURVIVAL SKILL 4
Time management and caseload management
Training needs:
- Establish criteria for prioritizing patient care activities.
- Develop mechanics for delegating care to supportive personnel.
- Cultivate skills in dove-tailing, grouping similar patients, and maximizing patient contact time.
- Assist with selection of appropriate patient education resources.
- Review criteria and the mechanism for referral to other team members.
- Develop the ability to prepare the patient for the next level of care.

SURVIVAL SKILL 5
Interacting with other health care professionals
Training needs:
- Develop effective strategies for communication, negotiation, and conflict resolution.
- Support in developing long-term working relationships with the team.
- Validate professional self-worth and patient advocacy skills.

SURVIVAL SKILL 6
Planning career development
Training needs:
- Validate acute care physical therapy practice as a viable long-term career option.
- Increase awareness of opportunities for professional growth and/or specialization within the acute care field.
- Develop networking skills internal and external to the practice setting.

Reprinted with permission. Curtis KA, Martin T. Recruitment & retention. Rehab Management. 1991;4:69-77.

SUMMARY

The acute care setting was one of the first practice settings to experience the influence of prospective payment systems on health care delivery. Increased patient co-morbidity, short lengths of stay, and an emphasis on discharge planning characterize today's acute care physical therapy practice.

This chapter has presented some strategies that can be used by physical therapists to provide effective and efficient care in the acute care setting. Therapists who are able to collaborate with other providers and prioritize their time and efforts will be most successful in the acute care setting. Strong patient and family education skills are essential to effective patient management. Development of these critical skills will serve physical therapists well in any practice setting.

REFERENCES

1. Curtis KA, Martin T. Perceptions of acute care physical therapy practice: issues for physical therapist preparation. *Phys Ther.* 1993;73(9):581-598.
2. Welch E, Anastasas M. Critical care, critical choices. *PT-Magazine of Physical Therapy.* 1996;4(3):75-77.
3. Woods EN. PTs in critical care. *PT-Magazine of Physical Therapy.* 1997;5(2):30-39.
4. Curtis KA, Martin T. Recruitment & retention. *Rehab Management.* 1991;4(5):69-70, 72, 74-76.
5. Arthur PR. Patient-focused care: Acute orthopedic services. *PT-Magazine of Physical Therapy.* 1994;2(7):33-47.
6. Reynolds JP. LOS:SOS. *PT-Magazine of Physical Therapy.* 1996;4(2):38-42,44-46.
7. *House of Delegates Policies; Position on Multi-skilled Personnel, HOD 06-95-27-17 (Program 32).* Alexandria, Va: American Physical Therapy Association; 1995.

TEST YOUR SKILLS

1. Name seven strategies that can be used by physical therapists in the acute care setting to maximize effectiveness and efficiency.
    1.
    2.
    3.
    4.
    5.
    6.
    7.

2. Name five factors that have influenced physical therapy practice in the acute care setting.
    1.
    2.
    3.
    4.
    5.

3. Name two reasons for hospital restructuring.
    1.
    2.

4. Name seven common characteristics of patient-focused care.
    1.
    2.
    3.
    4.
    5.
    6.
    7.

CHECK YOUR RESPONSES

1. Name seven strategies that can be used by physical therapists in the acute care setting.
    1. Utilize support personnel
    2. Utilize time-management techniques
    3. Group treatments
    4. Referring patients to nursing or restorative aides when skilled physical therapy is no longer needed
    5. Team conferences
    6. Critical pathways
    7. Chart by exception

2. Name five factors that have influenced physical therapy practice in the acute care setting.
    1. Patients with multiple diagnoses (co-morbidity)
    2. Older, sicker population
    3. Advances in modern medicine
    4. Decreased length of stay
    5. Hospital restructuring

3. Name two reasons for hospital restructuring.
    1. Cost containment
    2. To provide services in a way likely to increase patient satisfaction

4. Name seven common characteristics of patient-focused care.
    1. Grouping of patients with similar diagnoses and resource needs
    2. Decentralization of ancillary services
    3. Cross-training of employees to produce multi-skilled workers
    4. Transdisciplinary team approach
    5. Governance restructuring
    6. Critical pathways or care paths
    7. Charting by exception

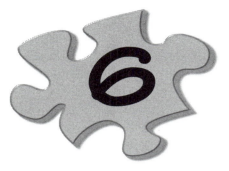

TRENDS & STRATEGIES FOR PHYSICAL THERAPY PRACTICE IN SUB-ACUTE CARE

Julie Roberson, MPT

Since managed care first burst onto the scene, we have seen many changes in the health care system. Perhaps the most dramatic changes have been related to the increased drive to cut health care costs. There is constant pressure to provide services at a lower rate than the competition. One way in which health care organizations are providing care at a lower cost is by offering sub-acute care, a setting that has seen rapid growth in recent years.

WHAT IS SUB-ACUTE CARE?

The Joint Commission on Accreditation of Healthcare Organizations (JCAHO) defines sub-acute care in this way:

> Sub-acute care is comprehensive inpatient care designed for someone who has had an acute illness, injury, or exacerbation of a disease process... Generally, the individual's condition is such that the care does not depend heavily on high technology monitoring or complex diagnostic procedures. It requires the coordinated services of an interdisciplinary team... Sub-acute care is generally more intensive than traditional nursing facility care and less than acute care...[1]

There is still some confusion as to what is included under the umbrella of sub-acute care. What types of facilities are considered sub-acute? What types of patients are seen there? To fully answer these questions, one must first understand the differences between the many settings within sub-acute care and outside its boundaries. Let's look at the differences between each of the following settings:

- Acute care hospitals
- Acute care rehabilitation
- Skilled nursing facilities
- Transitional care units
- Nursing homes

Acute care is usually well understood; it provides care to the more critically ill patient who, under the JCAHO definition, requires "high technology monitoring and complex diagnostic procedures." The typical patient in this setting remains hospitalized for an average of 5 days.[2] *Acute care rehabilitation*, on the other hand, is set up for patients with an intense need for rehabilitative services and who can handle 3 or 4 hours of therapy per day.[1] The average length of stay in this setting is 28 days.[3]

Under the realm of sub-acute care is the *skilled nursing facility* (SNF), which offers daily skilled nursing care or skilled rehabilitation services plus other medical services. SNFs provide necessary medical and 24-hour nursing care for the patient who does not require the specialized care of an acute hospital. Average length of stay in an SNF is 24 days.[3]

A variation of an SNF is the transitional care concept. Facilities are often known as *transitional care centers* (TCC) or *transitional care units* (TCU). Regardless of the name, it is essentially a "step-down" transitional setting used

Mrs. Beckwith was a 50-year-old schoolteacher who lived alone and was very active. One day when she was cleaning the rain gutters on her house, she fell off the ladder and fractured her hip. She was taken to Lakeside Hospital, where she underwent surgery to repair the fracture. Physical therapy treatment began the following day, but Mrs. Beckwith was suffering from excruciating pain. Three days later, she had managed to take a few steps with a walker but was still having difficulty with her pain. The doctors had a dilemma: Mrs. Beckwith was medically stable and no longer needed the advanced medical services the acute care hospital had to offer, but she was not ready to go home by herself. Luckily, the hospital also had a transitional care center, which would offer the same rehabilitation services but not the same medical services, which Mrs. Beckwith did not need anyway. She was transferred there that afternoon, and 5 days later she was able to go home.

by many hospitals to allow their patients to stay for a longer period of time before being discharged to home or to an extended care facility.

The idea of a TCU is being used more and more frequently by acute care hospitals. Such a unit was implemented in 1988 at Cedars Sinai Medical Center in Los Angeles. According to Carol Dobashi, PT, service line manager, the Skilled Nursing Assessment Center (SNAC) was developed "because we had a large orthopedic population at Cedars being discharged from the acute side, but they weren't quite ready for rehab yet." She went on to say that "(the patients) require some skilled help before they can go home, such as skilled nursing and therapies. They don't fit the traditional spinal cord, head trauma, cerebrovascular accident model that you'd see on the inpatient rehab unit, but they also don't belong on the acute care side anymore because their condition has stabilized."[1] The average length of stay for SNAC patients is 10 days, and 80% of these patients are discharged to home.[1]

Another sub-acute care setting is the *nursing home*. This term is sometimes used interchangeably with SNF and, in many ways, is very similar. The main difference between a SNF and a nursing home can be considered to be the level of care required by the patients. Generally speaking, a SNF offers nursing and rehabilitation services that are meant to improve and restore function, whereas a nursing home can be considered to provide custodial care and rehabilitation services to maintain a current level of function. Yet, many health care providers choose to label nursing homes as long-term care facilities.

A *long-term care facility* offers custodial care to residents unable to care for themselves and who do not have family members capable of caring for them. According to John Herringer of the JCAHO Standards Interpretation Department, the difference between sub-acute care and long-term care is the following: "Subacute care requires that at least an RN level of skill expertise be available on every unit on every shift, whereas a long-term care facility does not."[1]

THE GROWTH OF SUB-ACUTE CARE

Although sub-acute care has been around for many years, it was in the late 1980s that this setting saw drastic growth and changes. Most of this was related to changes in the Medicare system as influenced by new legislation at that time. The most significant was the passage of the Medicare Catastrophic Coverage Act. This changed the SNF provisions of that time by removing a 3-day hospital stay criterion, increasing coverage of SNF days from 100 to 150, eliminating the episode-of-illness concept and changing copayment structure.[4,6] This encouraged many facilities to seek out Medicare certification

TABLE 6.1					
Personal Health Care Expenditures (PHCE) and Distribution of Nursing Home Care Expenditures					
Year	PHCE in billions of dollars	Total nursing in billions of dollars	% PHCE	Medicare amt in billions of dollars	Medicare % of nursing home expenditures
1970	64.9	4.9	7.6	0.2	4.1
1988	482.8	42.8	8.9	1.0	2.3
1989	529.9	47.7	9.0	3.8	8.0
1990	585.3	53.1	9.1	2.5	4.7
1991	660.2	59.9	9.1	2.7	4.5

Adapted from Helbing C, Cornelius ES. Skilled Nursing Facilities. Health Care Financing Review. Annual Supplement. *Washington DC: Health Care Financing Administration;1992.*

because of the potential increase in reimbursement. This act was repealed in 1989, just a year after its passage, but not before there was a quadrupling of SNF use during that time.[6] That year also saw the Medicare certification of 1624 new SNFs.[6] Medicare spending for sub-acute care stays also saw a significant rise at that time, as illustrated in Table 6.1.

Currently, Medicare (Part A) hospital insurance will only pay for SNF care if six specific conditions are met:

- The patient's condition requires daily skilled nursing or skilled rehabilitation services that can only be provided in an SNF.
- The beneficiary was in a hospital at least 3 consecutive days prior to SNF admittance.
- The beneficiary was admitted to an SNF within 30 days after leaving a hospital.
- The care in the SNF is for a condition that was treated in the hospital or is for one that arose in the SNF.
- A medical professional certifies that the beneficiary needs skilled nursing or skilled rehabilitation services on a daily basis.
- A Medicare intermediary does not disapprove the stay.[4]

Once these conditions are met, the SNF stay is covered fully by Medicare Part A for the first 20 days, then covered at a set rate per day for the 21st through 100th day, and not covered at all after 100 days per episode of illness.[4,5] An *episode of illness* is the period from when the patient first receives hospital services to when he or she has not been in a hospital or SNF for 60 consecutive days.[4]

FUTURE GROWTH IN SUB-ACUTE CARE

There continues to be a growing need for SNF care. It is expected that by the year 2030, the over-65 population will have doubled to 65 million, and these are the individuals who are more likely to require the extended services of a sub-acute care facility.[7] We can, therefore, assume that the number of patients requiring sub-acute care will also double unless medical advances negate the need for such care by that time.

This brings up the question of whether there are enough facilities to provide that care. Estimates indicate a need for only six units per 1 million people, yet at this point in time there are approximately 63 units per million patients, an obvious surplus.[8] Harry Ting, PhD, author of *Subacute Care: Analysis of the Market Opportunities & Competition,* sums it up by saying, "There's substantial room for growth, but if you look at the number of potential competitors out there, it far exceeds the need."[8] The potential for population growth combined with the potential for increased revenue continues to fuel the growth of the sub-acute market. There is currently an estimated $3.4 billion in revenues generated annually in sub-acute care, and that figure is predicted to rise to $9.4 billion by the year 2000.[8] It is likely that as long as revenue is guaranteed, the number of sub-acute facilities will continue to rise.

COST CONTAINMENT AS RELATED TO SUB-ACUTE CARE

As the health care environment looks for more cost-cutting measures and as hospitals strive to repackage themselves, subacute care has emerged as the alternative to acute care[1]

Cost as related to sub-acute care is an ever-present issue. It's no secret that it is less expensive to receive care at a SNF than at a hospital. It is estimated that sub-acute care facilities can provide the same amount of care for 40% to 60% less than hospitals. This could compute into a cost savings of nearly $9 billion per year for Medicare alone, not to mention the potential savings to other programs.[7] Average daily charges in a sub-acute unit range from $300 to $550 per day, compared with $700 to $1000 at an acute care rehabilitation unit.[9]

Cost is not the only difference that can be found between sub-acute care and acute rehabilitation. In a study published in 1995, a comparison was made between the rehabilitation for a stroke patient in these two settings. The results are presented in Tables 6.2 through 6.4.

The main differences found between the two settings were length of stay,

TABLE 6.2

AVERAGE DAILY BILLED TREATMENT HOURS

Discipline	Acute rehab	Sub-acute rehab
Physical therapy	1.67*	.86
Occupational therapy	1.63*	.86
Speech therapy	.88	.90
Social service	.33*	.00
Psychology	.30*	.00
Other	.12*	.00
Average per day	4.92*	2.62
Average total hours	114.23*	50.66

*P <0 .0001 (t test, two-tailed)

Reprinted with permission from Keith RA, Wilson DB, Gutierrez P. Acute and subacute rehabilitation for stroke: a comparison. Arch Phys Med Rehabil. 1995;76:495-500.

TABLE 6.3

PRINCIPAL PAYMENT SOURCE

Payment source	Acute rehab		Sub-acute rehab	
	No.	%	No.	%
Medicare/Medicaid	207	62.5	37	38.1
Fee-for-service	33	10.0	2	2.1
Discounted contracts	27	8.2	8	8.2
Per diem rate	54	16.3	49	50.5
Other	10	3.0	1	1.0
Total	331	100.0	97	100.0

Reprinted with permission from Keith RA, Wilson DB, Gutierrez P. Acute and subacute rehabilitation for stroke: a comparison. Arch Phys Med Rehabil. 1995;76:495-500.

TABLE 6.4

DISCHARGE DESTINATION

Destination	Acute rehab		Sub-acute rehab	
	No.	%	No.	%
Residential setting	235	71.0	65	67.0
Nursing home	33	10.0	17	17.5
Acute care hospital	22	6.6	11	11.3
Other	41	12.4	4	4.1
Total	331	100.0	97	100.0

Reprinted with permission from Keith RA, Wilson DB, Gutierrez P. Acute and subacute rehabilitation for stroke: a comparison. Arch Phys Med Rehabil. 1995;76:495-500.

total billed hours for rehabilitative services, cost, and discharge destination. The average length of stay for the acute rehabilitation patient was 28.6 days, whereas for sub-acute it was 24.2 days. The total billed hours per patient was 114 hours for acute rehabilitation and 51 hours for sub-acute. This computes to approximately 5 hours per day of treatment for acute rehabilitation compared to 2 hours per day for sub-acute.

This means that the acute rehabilitation patient was receiving more than twice as many hours of rehabilitative services than the sub-acute patient. The costs reflected this increase in services with an average daily charge for acute rehabilitation of $1021 and an average for sub-acute of $502.[3]

According to this study, the differences in cost between these two settings is tremendous, yet this does not compute to a real difference between the outcome of the patients seen there. As reflected in the patients' scores on a Functional Independence Measure, the acute rehabilitation patients did have a higher total score at discharge than did the sub-acute patients, but this was not found by the researchers to be statistically significant. Based on this, one could consider that sub-acute care is simply a cost-efficient way to provide the same type of care as acute rehabilitation.

QUALITY OF CARE

Not everyone agrees that sub-acute care is offering the highest level of care possible. It is a major issue that has been repeatedly addressed by many involved. This can be discussed in two different ways: first by addressing the appropriateness of the level of care for the acuity of patients, and second by addressing the staffing available to provide that care and their qualifications to perform the tasks they are assigned.

Acuity of Patients

The overwhelming consensus concerning sub-acute care is that the acuity of patients is constantly increasing. Acute care hospitals tend to discharge patients sooner due to the ever-increasing emphasis on cost containment.[10] Because the patients aren't necessarily recovering sooner and subsequently being discharged to home, the next logical place to send them is the more cost-effective sub-acute care facility.

However, earlier discharge also means that the patient will be arriving at the sub-acute care facility with a greater acuity level, thereby requiring an increased level of skilled care. Mor, Banaszak-Holl, and Zinn noticed a trend toward specialization of skilled nursing facilities. They state that the "level of

TABLE 6.5

PERCENTAGE OF FACILITIES WITH TWO OR MORE PHYSICAL THERAPISTS ON STAFF (BY FACILITY SIZE: 1992 - 1995)

	1992	1993	1994	1995
< 100 beds	3%	4%	4.5%	5%
100+ beds	8%	8%	9%	13%

Adapted from Mor V, Banaszak-Holl J, Zinn J. The trend toward specialization in nursing care facilities. Generations. 1995-1996; 24-29.

intensity of medical and skilled nursing services provided in nursing care facilities has increased dramatically over the past decade."[11]

Staffing of Sub-acute Care Facilities

If the level of acuity of patients has increased in recent years, then one would assume that more staff, as well as more skilled workers, would need to be available to care for those patients. In the realm of physical therapy, this seems to be the case. One study reported the percentage of facilities with at least two full-time equivalent therapists on staff between 1992 and 1995 steadily increase (Table 6.5).[11]

This may not be the case in other professions, such as nursing, however. Roth and Harrison found that staff members of sub-acute care facilities were finding the acuity of their patients increasing but were not seeing their salaries increase accordingly, and in some cases, salaries even lagged behind those in acute care facilities.[10] This was noted to lead to a high turnover rate of professionals and, in turn, an inadequate presence of skilled employees for the level of acuity of patients.[10] Although no studies are noted to show this trend in physical therapy, this may be a source of concern for workers in this area and should undoubtedly be studied and monitored further.

REIMBURSEMENT ISSUES AND RECENT TRENDS

As salary is an issue for employees of sub-acute care facilities, the underlying financial problems can be traced back to the reimbursement of the facility for the services provided. With all the positive sides to the cost efficiency of these facilities, one would think that there would be no hesitation to pay for services provided there. Yet, this does not seem to be the case.

Most skilled nursing facility patients are elderly and eligible for Medicare coverage. Medicare, therefore, seems to have the major influence on reimbursement policy for skilled nursing facilities. Currently, there are drastic changes occurring with Medicare payment systems.

The current trend in health care is to switch to a prospective payment system (PPS) for reimbursement. This involves determining an amount to pay out to a provider in advance that is intended to cover a number of items and services.[13] The reason for doing this is simple: spending for sub-acute care has risen dramatically over the past few years and is projected to continue on this trend.[4] Action to halt this growth led to the initiation of a prospective payment system for skilled nursing facilities.[14,15]

PROSPECTIVE PAYMENT SYSTEM FOR SKILLED NURSING FACILITIES

The Balanced Budget Act of 1997 introduced changes to the Medicare system that affect skilled nursing facility coverage. In mid-1998, skilled nursing facilities began the transition to a PPS for their Part A inpatient services. These PPS payments are based on per-diem rates and cover all costs of furnishing covered SNF services, including routine, ancillary, and capital-related costs.[16]

It is important to note that the PPS for SNFs is different from PPS diagnosis-related groups (DRGs) for acute hospitals. SNF PPS is based on the intensity and complexity of services given to the patient, while PPS for acute hospitals is based on the diagnosis and age of the patient.[16]

OUTCOMES EVALUATION

Physical therapists may be greatly affected by the current trends and changes in the sub-acute care setting. For this reason, physical therapists must take a pro-active role to ensure that the policies created within the changing system will best reflect the desires and wishes of the physical therapy profession. As this issue is addressed, the question arises in regard to which method of intervention is most appropriate. An example of a method currently being used is *outcomes evaluation.*

This is a method to measure the effectiveness and efficiency of achievement of results, as well as customer satisfaction.[17] By monitoring these factors, therapists can provide statistics and data as related to quality of care in order to help strengthen their stand when dealing with any undesired situations that might arise within the sub-acute care setting. According to Steve Forer, president of Quality and Outcome Management in Hayward, Calif, some of the benefits of outcomes evaluation are "identification of problem areas requiring more detailed investigation, better alignment of goals and objectives with client needs, use of outcomes data for research purposes, and cost-effectiveness information."[17]

For a sub-acute facility to begin an outcomes evaluation program, one should understand more about it. There are three main types of outcomes assessments: *global*, *program-specific*, and *patient-specific*. *Global outcome assessment* involves the evaluation of diverse populations of patients for generalizations to be made regarding care. A common type would be the functional independence measure. The disadvantage of global assessment is that there is a low ability to reflect small changes in a specific area of function.

The second type of assessment, or *program-specific outcome assessment*, involves gathering information on select groups of rehabilitation patients who have similar functional limitations and similar treatment programs. This is useful in evaluating the effectiveness of a specific treatment.

The third type of outcome assessment is the *patient-specific outcome assessment*, which is used to evaluate the effectiveness of a patient's rehabilitation program in meeting his or her goals. This method is the most specific but least generalizable.[18]

After the different types of outcome assessments are understood, it is then important to identify the caseload composition, impairments, and diagnostic groups.[17] Outcomes should then be measured at discharge and 6 to 9 months after discharge.[16] Facilities often have research experts who supervise the gathering of these data or should consider this approach.[18] As these data are collected and analyzed, sub-acute facilities can get a clearer view of where they stand on issues of quality of care and cost efficiency. By learning this information sooner, they can then make the appropriate adjustments needed to have a firm hold in today's health care system.

SUMMARY

As with all other aspects of health care, the sub-acute care setting has changed drastically in recent years and continues to do so. Through careful inspection of this setting, one can see that there are many positive points to its utilization, especially when considering cost efficiency. The care provided has proven to be adequate and similar to that provided in an acute rehabilitation setting with regard to patient outcome. It would seem, therefore, that there are no inadequacies with this setting. Yet, the recent changes in the reimbursement issues for sub-acute care have caused physical therapists to become alarmed and to take notice of the changes to come. This will be an area closely watched in the coming years, and we can hope that a balance will be met between all aspects and all parties involved.

REFERENCES

1. Monahan B. Subacute care: a new or old continuum? *PT-Magazine of Physical Therapy.* 1996;4(2):30-37.
2. Reynolds JP. LOS: SOS. *PT-Magazine of Physical Therapy.* 1996;4(2):38-46.
3. Keith RA, Wilson DB, Gutierrez P. Acute and subacute rehabilitation for stroke: a comparison. *Arch Phys Med Rehabil.* 1995;76:495-500.
4. Helbing C, Cornelius ES. Chapter 5: Skilled nursing facilities. *Health Care Financing Review.* 1992 Annual Supplement:97-123.
5. Bodenheimer TS, Grumbach K. *Understanding Health Policy: A Clinical Approach.* Stamford, CT: Appleton and Lange; 1995.
6. Manton KG, Stallard E, Woodbury MA. Home health and skilled nursing facility use: 1982-90. *Health Care Financing Review.* 1994;16(1):155-186.
7. Cleary A. The long view on long-term care. *Hospitals & Health Networks.* 1995; 69(6):61-62,64.
8. Lumsdon K. Like ants to a picnic. *Hospitals & Health Networks.* 1995;69(10):47.
9. Tokarski C. Riding the express: is your subacute strategy on track? *Hospitals & Health Networks.* 1995:69(3):20-23.
10. Roth PA, Harrison JK. Ethical conflict in long-term care: is legislation the answer? *J Prof Nurs.* 1994;10(5):271-277.
11. Mor V, Banaszak-Holl J, Zinn J. The trend toward specialization in nursing care facilities. *Generations.* 1995-1996;Winter:24-29.
12. Cohn R. Managed care in intermediate settings part II: selection and implementation of a contract. *PT-Magazine of Physical Therapy.* 1996;4(9):20-23.
13. Grotch GR. Prospective payment systems for post acute care. *PT-Magazine of Physical Therapy.* 1997;5(4):14-16.
14. Olsen GG, Jenson JI. New payment system for SNFs. *Rehab Management.* 1996;9(1):101-103.
15. Phillips P. Medicare strategies group formulates PPS recommendations. *PT-Magazine of Physical Therapy.* 1997;5(2):10-11, 19.
16. *The Balanced Budget Act—How it Affects Physical Therapy.* Alexandria, Va: American Physical Therapy Association, http://www.apta.org/govt_aff/bbasynop.html#II. Skilled Nursing Facilities, 6/28/98.
17. Forer S. Outcomes evaluation in subacute care. *Rehab Management.* 1995;8(4):138-140, 164.
18. Moore RW, Salcido R. Rehabilitation outcomes in subacute care. *Rehab Management.* 1996;9(1):97-98, 111.

TEST YOUR SKILLS

1. Define three types of sub-acute care facilities and differentiate them from acute care hospitals and acute care rehabilitation.
2. What caused a drastic increase in SNF use in the late 1980s?
3. What are the implications of prospective payment systems on physical therapy services in skilled nursing facilities?
4. What are three types of outcomes assessments?

CHECK YOUR RESPONSES

1. **Define three types of sub-acute care facilities and differentiate them from acute care hospitals and acute care rehabilitation.**
    1. Skilled nursing facilities
    2. Transitional care units
    3. Nursing homes

Acute care provides care to the more critically ill patient who requires high-technology monitoring and complex diagnostic procedures. The typical patient in this setting remains for an average of 5 days.

Acute care rehabilitation, on the other hand, is set up for patients with an intense need for rehabilitative services and who can handle 3 or 4 hours of therapy per day. The average length of stay for this setting is 28 days.

2. **What caused a drastic increase in SNF use in the late 1980s?**

The Medicare Catastrophic Coverage Act.

This changed the SNF provisions of that time by removing a 3-day hospital stay criterion, increasing coverage of SNF days from 100 to 150, eliminating the episode-of-illness concept, and changing copayment structure. This encouraged many facilities to seek out Medicare certification because of the potential increase in reimbursement. This act was repealed in 1989, just a year after its passage, but not before there was a quadrupling of SNF use and Medicare certification of 1624 new facilities during that time.

3. **What are the implications of prospective payment systems on physical therapy services in skilled nursing facilities?**

Prior to the implementation of a prospective payment system, physical therapy services provided in an SNF were billed to a Medicare intermediary on a reduced fee-for-service basis. In contrast, the newly instituted PPS payments are based on per-diem rates and cover all costs of furnishing covered SNF services, including routine, ancillary, and capital-related costs.

Physical therapy services will, therefore, be a cost center, rather than a revenue-generating entity, in the SNF and will be covered from this per-diem rate. Efficient and cost-effective physical therapy care will be even more valued as the financial impact of these changes become evident.

4. **What are three types of outcomes assessments?**
    1. Global
    2. Program-specific
    3. Patient-specific

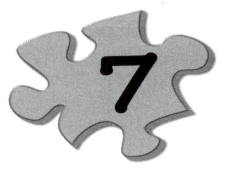

TRENDS & STRATEGIES FOR PHYSICAL THERAPY PRACTICE IN HOME HEALTH CARE

Nichole Hodson-Chennault, MPT

Home health care is one of the fastest growing areas of the health care industry. Cost-containment issues have led to the decreased length of stay in acute hospitals and increased use of skilled nursing facilities. Because of the push for discharge, patients are leaving the acute care setting with multiple problems and are less able to care for themselves. This has increased the delivery of services in the home.

Mr. Mack, at age 70, had a right total hip replacement (THR) 2 days ago. His insurance company paid the hospital a per-episode rate for Mr. Mack's stay. To contain costs, the hospital tries to discharge all patients with THR insured by XYZ Insurance within 3 to 5 days. His insurance coverage provides for home health care if medically necessary. Upon discharge from the hospital, he was able to ambulate 20 feet with a front-wheeled walker, and he required minimal assistance in his transfers. He went home with his 60-year-old wife. His doctor prescribed home health care for dressing changes, monitoring of his anti-coagulant therapy, and rehabilitative care.

DEFINITION OF HOME HEALTH CARE

Home health care encompasses a wide range of health and social services delivered in the homes of recovering, disabled, and chronically or terminally ill people in need of medical, nursing, social, or therapeutic treatment and/or assistance with the essential activities of daily living. Home care includes the provision of equipment and services to the patient in the home for the purposes of restoring and maintaining his or her maximal level of comfort, function, safety, and health.[1,2]

After evaluating Mr. Mack, the physical therapist determined that home safety equipment, such as a transfer bench and grab bars for the shower, an elevated toilet seat, patient education on area rugs and adequate lighting, as well as instruction on therapeutic exercises, was necessary for the safety of this patient.

BENEFITS OF RECEIVING HOME CARE

From the patient's point of view, home care seems to be the most efficient, effective, and least traumatic form of medical care, resulting in increased patient dignity and comfort. Additionally, when patients feel more comfortable in their homes, they have an increased level of motivation and sense of control.

These feelings of control may help to decrease patient anxiety and depression, helping to create active participation and enhancing the healing process. Generally, people recover more quickly at home rather than in the hospital. The quality of life for elderly people who remain in the community and receive care in the home is consistently better than those who enter long-term care facilities.[3]

Many studies have stressed the importance of the family and social support network in the functional recovery of elderly patients. The involvement of the patient, as well as his or her family, in his or her treatment program is one of the factors that lead to the enhancement of therapeutic effectiveness that is the hallmark of home care today.[1]

Additional advantages of home care:
- Privacy—Personal care in the home.
- Convenience—No transportation problems, less disruption of schedules.
- Lower costs—The costs of home care are much lower than care in a hospital or long-term care facility.
- Cost coverage—Medicare and Medicaid, as well as private insurance, usually cover medically necessary home care.
- Increased quality of life—Patients receiving home care generally report a greater sense of dignity and social interaction.

RECIPIENTS OF HOME CARE

Home care is one of the fastest growing areas in health care. This trend is fueled by the explosive growth of the elderly population older than 65.[4] Generally, elderly recipients of home care have experienced functional limitations in one or more of their activities of daily living or have just been discharged from a hospital stay.

Geriatric patients, however, are not the only recipients of home care. Children and adults who are disabled or chronically ill may require home medical services, such as nursing or physical therapy, to treat active problems and restore function. For example, younger adults and chronically ill children who experience disabling diseases such as multiple sclerosis or muscular dystrophy may benefit from home care. Adults and children diagnosed with illnesses, such as cancer or AIDS, also receive home care.

HOME HEALTH CARE PROVIDERS

Hospital-based Home Care

Efforts to improve continuity of care have led to an increase in hospital-based home care. *Hospital-based home care* refers to a hospital that provides its own home care services, rather than contracting with or referring to an external home health agency. This allows the hospital to manage a patient's care more comprehensively across the service continuum.

Home Health Agencies

Home health agencies are defined by their regulators as public or private agencies or organizations primarily engaged in providing skilled nursing or other therapeutic services.[5] These agencies are highly supervised and controlled (ie, by the Joint Commission on Accreditation of Healthcare Organizations or Accreditation Commission for Home Care, Inc). Some agencies deliver a variety of care through physicians, nurses, therapists, social workers, and homemakers, while others limit their services to only nursing. Patients requiring skilled home care services usually receive their care from a home health agency.

The term *home health agency* usually indicates that a home care provider is Medicare certified. A Medicare-certified agency has met federal minimum requirements for patient care and management and, therefore, can provide Medicare and Medicaid home health services.[1]

Home Health Registries

Home health registries are not home health agencies. Registries serve as employment agencies for home care nurses and aides by matching these providers with clients and collecting finders fees.[1] They are not required to screen the caregivers or to do background checks. The patient selects and supervises the caregiver, as well as pays the provider directly out of his or her pocket.

Hospice

Hospice services are available to individuals who are terminally ill and have a life expectancy of 6 months or less. Services are covered by Medicare. Hospice care involves an interdisciplinary team of health care providers and volunteers who provide medical care, as well as psychological and spiritual care, for the terminally ill. They also provide support for the patients' families. Care includes the provision of related medications, medical supplies, and equipment. It is based primarily in the home, allowing families to stay together.

MEDICAL TEAM MEMBERS PROVIDING HOME HEALTH CARE

Ralph was a 76-year-old man who had struggled with medical problems ranging from a stroke to digestive problems for the past 8 years. Three months ago, he was diagnosed with pancreatic cancer. Rather than have his last days spent in a hospital, he and his wife chose to have him spend his final days in the comfort of his home. As the end grew closer, he entered hospice care. The hospice health care provider administered an intravenous morphine drip to help ease his pain. She also provided emotional support for Ralph's family.

Physician

The physician usually acts as a gatekeeper for the delivery of home care. Physicians are initial contacts when entering the health care system. The physician makes referrals, receives the care reports, and must authorize the home health services provided. They ensure that all treatments rendered will be appropriate and in the best interest of the patient. Physicians may also visit the patients directly in the home to diagnose and treat illnesses.

Physical Therapist

The 1995 American Physical Therapy Association (APTA) membership survey reported that physical therapy was the third most regularly used type of home health care service.[6] A model definition of physical therapy is "the assessment, evaluation, treatment, and prevention of physical disability, movement dysfunction, and pain resulting from injury, disease, disability, or other health-related conditions."[7] Physical therapists work to restore strength and mobility, as well as prevent further dysfunction of patients who are home bound. Implied in the status of "home bound" is the requirement that the patient is not able to get out and function independently. Researchers have documented the finding that strength training can improve the mobility and function of the frail elderly.[8]

Physical therapists who work in home care may set goals to improve the patients' functional level in the home and community, implement pain management techniques, as well as instruct the patient in therapeutic exercises to improve strength, endurance, and range of motion. Additionally, home health physical therapists are ideal in enhancing the safety of their patients by identifying hazards and modifying the environment. Unfortunately, approximately one-third of the elderly fall each year, and one-third of those falls are attributed to environmental hazards.[6] Physical therapists can help prevent unnecessary falls and, in turn, debilitating injuries.

In today's health care system, patients are leaving the hospital with more acute conditions and less independence in their own care and mobility. With increased acuity, physical therapists now must have an even higher level of clinical judgment, as they may be the only health care provider making regular contact with the patient.

Physical therapists assume the role of the primary caregiver for many patients in the home health care setting. Not only do physical therapists focus on physical functioning and mobility, but they must also be aware of patient needs that go beyond the traditional physical therapy role. For example, although medication management is usually performed by nurses, physical therapists also monitor the use of medication by the questions they ask and the symptoms they observe during treatment sessions.[4]

Physical therapists providing home care use a range of clinical decision-making skills. Unlike therapists working in clinics, those working in home care do not have the advantage of working in close proximity to other therapists.[6] Because home health physical therapists practice in an independent environment, evaluation skills, judgment, and technical skills must be well-developed.[7] Home care physical therapists need the skills and knowledge base of both acute and rehabilitation therapists. They must have high-level screening and diagnostic skills to identify patient problems requiring immediate medical intervention.

Nikki, a new graduate physical therapist, has just signed on with ABC Home Health Agency. In her second week on the job, she was sent out to evaluate a patient who had a right total knee replacement 1 week earlier. Upon arriving at the home, Nikki noticed that the continuous passive motion machine was not positioned correctly and that the patient's right foot was excessively swollen. The patient reported that he was not able to move his ankle. Upon evaluation, Nikki found that the patient had impaired sensation, an absent pedal pulse, and a positive Homan's sign. The patient was also hypertensive and diaphoretic. Nikki called the patient's physician and reported the findings before proceeding with the care of this patient. The patient was admitted a few hours later to an acute hospital and treated for deep venous thrombosis.

Physical Therapist Assistant

The physical therapist assistant (PTA) works under the ongoing supervision of a licensed physical therapist. Once the physical therapist conducts an evaluation of a patient, the PTA may provide ongoing care. The PTA may perform skilled procedures and related tasks that have been selected and delegated by the supervising physical therapist.[9]

Registered Nurse

Nurses provide skilled services including patient assessments, designing care plans, administering medications by injection and intravenous therapy, wound care, and education on disease treatment and prevention. Nurses are often involved in monitoring chronic conditions and providing periodic reassessments of the patient's condition.

Home Health Aide

Home health aides generally have a high school education and on-the-job training to provide personal care services, such as bathing, dressing, and grooming activities. They also check vital signs, help with simple prescribed exercises, and assist with medication routines. Occasionally, they change nonsterile dressings, use special equipment, and assist with exercises or ambulation.[10]

Homemaker home health aides provide housekeeping services, personal care, and emotional support for their clients.[10] They clean clients' houses, do laundry, and change bed linens. Aides may also plan meals (including special diets), shop for food, and cook.

In home health agencies, home health aides are supervised by a registered nurse, a physical therapist, or a social worker who assigns them specific duties. Aides report changes in the client's condition to the supervisor or case manager.[10]

Social Worker

Social workers evaluate the social and emotional factors affecting the patient. They may provide counseling and referrals as needed. Social workers also work with the patient and family to identify community services that are available to the patient.

Occupational Therapist

The occupational therapist focuses on deficits in activities of daily living, such as adaptive feeding, dressing, grooming, bathing, and homemaking skills. In contrast, the physical therapist is usually more concerned with mobility activities, such as ambulation, transfers, and bed mobility. The two roles often overlap and complement each other.

Other Professions Providing Home Health Care

Other professionals who may be involved in the care of a patient include speech and language pathologists (SLPs), dietitians, and respiratory therapists. The severity of the patient's needs will determine what type of intervention is indicated.

GROWTH TRENDS IN HOME HEALTH CARE

Cost Effectiveness

When the costs of acute hospital care and SNF care are compared to the costs of home health care, home health care is by far the most cost-effective alternative (Table 7.1).

When comparing the various disciplines of care, it is evident that the costs of home care have risen in the past decade (Table 7.2). However, it is still much less expensive when compared to either acute hospital care or SNF care.

TABLE 7.1

COMPARISON OF HOSPITAL, SNF, AND HOME HEALTH CARE MEDICARE CHARGES, 1993 - 1996[11]

	1993	1994	1995	1996
Hospital charges per day	$1617	$1756	$1810	$1872
SNF charges per day	$305	$313	$323	$334
Home care charges per visit	**$81**	**$83**	**$86**	**$88**

TABLE 7.2

AVERAGE COSTS PER HOME CARE VISIT BY VARIOUS HOME HEALTH CARE PERSONNEL: 1987 - 1996[11]

	1987	1996
Nurse	$62	$99
Physical therapist	$57	$91
Home care aide	$34	$55
Homemaker	$33	$52

Employment Opportunities

With the apparent cost effectiveness of home health care, it is no surprise that this industry is one of the fastest growing areas of health care. With this growth comes increased employment opportunities. In the past, many physical therapists just moonlighted as home health providers to make "extra cash." However, many are now working in home care full-time. Current APTA statistics indicate that out of 40,194 member physical therapists, 9.9% work in the home health setting, while out of 4740 PTAs, 7.4% are currently working in home health care.[12] The total number of home care employees has risen to serve the increased demand of home care services. Between 1991 and 1995, home care employment grew from 344,000 to 610,000 employees, at an average rate of 15% per year[11] (Table 7.3).

Hospital-based Home Care

Hospital-based home care agencies have grown faster than any other type of certified agency. Since 1980, there has been an 11.5% increase in hospital-based home care agencies.[11] Hospitals that operate home care programs have received an add-on to Medicare's cost-based reimbursement for home care to cover their additional overhead expenses. This incentive may be related to the increase in these types of services, as discharge to a hospital-based home care

TABLE 7.3

TOTAL EMPLOYMENT IN HOME HEALTH CARE: 1991 - 1995[11,13]

Year	Number of employees
1991	344,000
1992	398,000
1993	469,000
1994	555,000
1995	610,000

TABLE 7.4

SOURCES OF PAYMENT FOR HOME HEALTH CARE: 1992 - 1994[11]

Source of payment	1992 home health care	1994 home health care
Medicare	37.8%	60.0%
Medicaid	24.7%	14.4%
Private insurance	5.5%	8.4%
Out-of-pocket	31.4%	3.1%
Other	0.6%	14.1%

program may alleviate some of the financial pressures imposed by per-episode reimbursement of the acute hospital stay. The potential for overutilization is present as well. According to the Department of Health and Human Services, 62% of patients discharged from hospitals that own a home health agency were referred to an agency owned by that hospital.[15]

Payers of Service and Reimbursement

Medicare is the largest single payer of home care services.[11,17] Table 7.4 illustrates the major sources of payment for home health care services.

Medicare Reimbursement

Part A Medicare coverage will pay for services provided by a home care agency that are deemed medically necessary only if <u>all</u> of the following conditions are met:

- The care included intermittent skilled nursing care, physical therapy, or speech therapy.
- The individual must be confined to the home (homebound).
- The individual must be under the care of a physician who determines that the individual needs home care and who set up the home care plan.

- The home care agency providing the covered services must be certified as a participant in the Medicare program.[17]
- Physical therapists must provide documentation that meets these Medicare guidelines if they expect their services to be reimbursed.

Medicare will pay for services if the services are "reasonable and necessary." *Reasonable care* means a greater-than-chance probability that a patient will make a significant improvement as a result of physical therapy services. A reasonable amount of time means that the planned frequency and duration of treatments established by the therapist are consistent with the patient's diagnosis. *Necessary* means that the services provided can only be safely and effectively performed by a physical therapist. See Chapter 11 for a more detailed description of documentation requirements.

Medicare will pay for physical therapy services that result in functional, sustainable, and measurable changes in a patient's condition or that significantly improve the patient's quality of life.[14] It will cover full reasonable costs of home care services as long as the service is medically necessary. If the services are not deemed necessary, clients of Medicare may be charged for the services that are not covered.

Medicaid

Medicaid is a joint federal-state medical assistance program offered to low-income individuals. Classified recipients include certain aged, blind, and/or disabled individuals who have incomes that are too high to qualify for mandatory coverage but are below federal poverty levels. Under federal Medicaid rules, coverage of home health services must include part-time nursing, home care aide services, and medical supplies and equipment. At the states' option, Medicaid may also cover physical therapy, occupational therapy, speech and language pathology, and medical social services.[1]

Medigap

Medicare insurance does not cover all health care expenses. Medigap insurance is designed to bridge the gap in Medicare coverage; it is a type of supplemental insurance for expenses not covered by Part B. Medigap policies offer at-home recovery benefits, which will pay for some personal care services when the patient is receiving Medicare-covered skilled home health care.

Private Insurance and Out-of-Pocket Payment

Private insurance can be either individual or employment-based. Many pri-

Mrs. Bruce was recently discharged from the hospital after having a left total knee replacement. Her physician decided that home health physical therapy was necessary for patient instruction on therapeutic exercise and safety education. Medicare covered all reasonable medical costs of her home therapy, including rental of a walker. During the last session of physical therapy, Mrs. Bruce asked her therapist if she could get her a wheelchair so she could go to church. She said the pews in her church were too low. Unfortunately, Medicare would not cover the cost of renting a wheelchair in addition to the other equipment she had already received. If Mrs. Bruce wanted the wheelchair, she would have to pay out of her own pocket. Mrs. Bruce could not afford to rent the wheelchair herself, so she watched a televised service for the next few weeks.

vate insurance policies cover home health with varying coverage limits. Additionally, some patients do not have any medical insurance coverage. These patients must pay for services directly.

The Balanced Budget Act of 1997 and Changes in Home Health Care

Currently, a variety of proposed changes to Medicare reimbursement for home health care are surfacing. The Balanced Budget Act of 1997 was signed into legislation on August 5, 1997. It created dramatic changes for Medicare home health care benefits. Cuts to home health care will total more than $115 billion over the next 5 years. Congress reports that these changes are needed to fight fraud and abuse and to keep Medicare from bankruptcy.[21]

Some changes specific to home health care

- Implemented home care agency cost limits are to be reduced. This change is estimated to reduce cost limits at least 7%.[22]
- A new prospective payment system (PPS) for home health agencies is to be implemented for cost periods beginning on or after October 1, 1999.[22-24] This PPS will involve per-episode reimbursement.
- A new per-beneficiary annual limit will be determined.[22]
- Not all home health care services will be covered under Part A. Only cases in which there was prior 3-day hospitalization will be covered. Additionally, coverage will be limited to 100 visits.[22-24] Home care reimbursement will then shift to Medicare Part B coverage after 100 visits or if no 3-day hospital stay precedes home care.

Further considerations

The above changes may deny needed home care services to millions of seniors and people with disabilities. What then? Health care providers must provide evidence to legislators that specific limitations to home care may compromise patient health and safety and lead to more costly institutional care at a later date.

Documentation and Reimbursement

Physical therapists need to document the patient's need for skilled physical therapy services and show objective measurable progress. Functional tools that have been tested for validity should be used to document a patient's status. Additionally, these tools should be practical, portable, and easy to use.[25] Some examples of functional assessment tools used by the physical therapist in a home health setting include the Tinetti Balance and Mobility Assessment, the Barthel Index, and the Timed Up-and-Go.[25,26]

To minimize the risk of denial for reimbursement, the following components should be included in patient documentation:

- Reason the patient is homebound
- Objective findings of the evaluation and progress made on re-evaluation
- Functional goals and timelines
- Treatment plan must be related to functional goals
- Home program instructions
- Safety hazards
- Plan for discharge from the first visit
- All conferences with all health care team members (ie, occupational therapy, PT, SLP, nursing, home health aide)

There are certain key words and phrases to avoid using, as they may lead to claim denials. For example, do not use the following terms:

- Patient is "stabilized" (if not planning to discharge)
- Patient is "doing well" (state what the patient has done to overcome his or her limitation)
- "Maintains" range of motion or strength
- Use arrows or terms such as increase or decrease without including specific objective measures (ie, increase from 20° flexion to 45° flexion)
- "Same" on each visit note

The above lists are not all inclusive; however, they should give the reader some guidelines for successful and informative documentation.[6] More detailed coverage of documentation requirements is included in Chapter 11.

Time Management and Cost Containment

A recent study found that physical therapists spend an average of 74 minutes per home heath visit.[6] With the field of home health growing and reimbursement changing to a PPS, it is important to develop strategies to help manage time and contain costs. Some strategies to help manage time are to see all patients in the same geographical area at one time. Additionally, it is important to receive clear, concise directions to the patient's house. Having pre-written educational materials and therapeutic equipment in the trunk of the car will also improve efficiency during the treatment session.

It is also beneficial to have a referral relationship with durable medical equipment suppliers in the area and to carry a pre-printed list of phone numbers. Medical equipment suppliers provide home care patients with products ranging from respirators to shower bars. These companies will usually deliver and set up the equipment, as well as instruct the patient on proper use.

Call first to verify patient coverage for medical equipment. Many third-party payers require prior authorization of equipment rental or purchase or may require services from a particular vendor. Additionally, there may be significant coverage restrictions that may influence therapist recommendations. For example, Medicare will not cover a high-rise toilet seat and a shower chair, but instead will authorize a "3-in-1 chair" to cover both needs. Similarly, Medicare restricts the rental of both a walker and a wheelchair.

Involving the patient's family in his or her home care can also increase therapist efficiency. First, it is important to educate the patient, as well as the family, on the purpose of physical therapy intervention. The family can be involved by completing a home evaluation checklist before the first evaluation session. The therapist and family can then review the checklist together, answer questions, and discuss any equipment recommendations or changes to the home structure that may be beneficial.

Consistent Communication

Consistent communication with the other health care team members can help improve the quality of care the patient receives by ensuring that all the professionals providing care are working toward the same goals. It is important to document both telephone communication and formal team conferences between team members. This will help to avoid miscommunication.

Susan Doe, PT, received a referral from Dr. Franklin to do an evaluation on a patient who had multiple problems. Prior to the evaluation day, Susan telephoned the patient to set an appointment time. She was able to speak with the patient's daughter, who was eager to participate in her mother's care. Susan arranged to fax the home checklist to the patient's daughter. The patient's daughter agreed to fill out the form that evening.

The home checklist asked questions like, "What equipment does the patient have?" (ie, walker, cane, crutches, gripper, commode) "What modifications or structural changes have been made to the home?" (ie, ramp, shower bars) "Are there night lights in the home? Are there area rugs?" When Susan arrived to conduct the evaluation, the daughter had the form completed. They reviewed the patient's needs together. This saved Susan approximately 20 minutes, so instead of making two visits to complete the initial evaluation, she only had to charge for one 50-minute evaluation. This form saved time and money!

SUMMARY

Physical therapists play an important role in patient care. With the field of home health rapidly growing, it is important to be prepared to be able to provide home health care to our patients. This involves high-level skills in evaluating and treating patients with multiple medical diagnoses, collaborating with other team members involved with the patient's care, considering the patient's payment source, as well as performing appropriate documentation to ensure reimbursement and quality care.

When a physical therapist enters the home to provide treatment for the patient, he or she is often the only health care provider present. Therapist evaluation skills, clinical decision-making skills, and treatment skills must be well-developed. The physical therapist must listen to, evaluate, and respond to patient concerns, communicating with the nurse or physician as necessary to inform him or her of the situation. As the field of home health care expands, so do our responsibilities as physical therapists.

REFERENCES

1. National Association for Home Care. *How to Choose a Home Care Provider.* http://www.nahc.org/Consumer/htcahca.html. 3/30/98.
2. Council on Scientific Affairs. Home care in the 1990s. *JAMA.* 1992;263(9):1241-1244.
3. Horizon Nursing Daycare. *Adult Day Care, a Sensible Solution.* http://home.algorithms.net/Horizon/frmain.htm, 3/30/98.
4. Young GJ. Home health: special risks. *PT-Magazine of Physical Therapy.* 1993;1(9):63-64.

5. May BJ. *Home Health and Rehabilitation, Concepts of Care*. Philadelphia: FA Davis Company; 1993.

6. Collins J, Beissner KL, Krout JA. Home health physical therapy: Practice patterns in western New York. *Magazine of Physical Therapy*. 1998;78(2):170-179.

7. Carr MN. We in home care; yesterday, today, & tomorrow. *Caring Magazine*. 1994;13(4):38-40.

8. Chandler JM, Duncan PW, Kochersberger G, Studenski S. Is lower extremity strength gain associated with improvement in physical performance and disability in frail, community-dwelling elders? *Arch Phys Med Rehabil*. 1998;79(1):24-30.

9. Section on Community Home Health, American Physical Therapy Association. *Guidelines for the Provision of Physical Therapy in the Home*. Alexandria, VA: American Physical Therapy Association, 1996.

10. US Department of Labor. Homemaker-Home Health Aides, in *1996-97 Occupational Outlook Handbook*. http://www.jobquest.com/ooh1996/ooh/ooh17201.htm, 3/30/98.

11. National Association for Home Care. *Basic Statistics about Home Care in 1996*. http://www.nahc.org/Consumer/hcstats.html. 3/30/98.

12. American Physical Therapy Association. *Demographic Description of Membership, 1997*. Alexandria, VA: American Physical Therapy Association; 1997. http://www.apta.org/research/pt_fac.html. 3/30/98.

13. American Physical Therapy Association. *Demographic Description of Affiliate Membership, 1997*. Alexandria, VA: American Physical Therapy Association; 1997. http://www.apta.org/research/pta_fac.html. 3/30/98.

14. Brittingham KM, Dempster M. Occupational therapists in home health care: ensuring positive outcomes through collaboration. *Occupational Therapists in Home Health Care*. 1990;2(1):32-44.

15. Many hospitals self-refer patients for home care services, HHS says. *PT Bulletin*. 1998;13(2):3, 6.

16. Anderson HJ. Hospital-based home care poised for growth in the 1990's. *Hospitals*. 1992;66(17):60-63.

17. Korenjak MF, Weinstein A. Medicare reimbursement for home care: past & future. *Caring Magazine*. 1996;15(3):30-34.

18. Bodenheimer TS, Grumbach K. *Understanding Health Policy, a Clinical Approach*. Stamford, Conn: Appleton & Lange; 1995.

19. Borger G. A magic Medicare moment. (Medicare legislation). *U.S. News & World Report*. 1997;123(1):36-38.

20. Wealthier beneficiaries pay more in Senate-Passed Medicare Reform. *PT Bulletin*. 1997;12(27):1, 12.

21. *The Home Health Crisis, a Special Series of In-depth Reports*. http://www. wksu.kent/news/stories/healthcare, 3/30/98.

22. California Association for Health Services at Home; News forum. *Budget Agreement Reached*. http://www.cahsah.org/budgetup.htm#top, 3/30/98.

23. Smith KT. Balanced Budget Act of 1997 becomes a reality: brings major changes to health care. *Nursing Economics*. 1997;15(5):271-274.

24. Center for Medicare Advocacy, Inc. *Balanced Budget Act of 1997 Creates Major Changes in the Medicare Home Health Program*. http://www.nsclc.org/hhlaw-sum.html, 3/30/98.

25. Moffa-Trotter M, Anemaet WK. Measuring up in home health; documenting objective, measurable progress in home care: two sample tools. *Advance/Rehabilitation*. 1995; 4(7):23-27.

26. Thompson M, Medley A. Performance of community dwelling elderly on the Timed Up and Go Test. *Physical & Occupational Therapy in Geriatrics*. 1995;13(3):17-30.

TEST YOUR SKILLS

Your mother has a history of hypertension and diabetes, and she is partially blind in her right eye. Until now, she has managed to live alone in her mobile home park. Five days ago, she slipped in her kitchen and fractured her hip. She had an open reduction and internal fixation 4 days ago to repair the fracture. The discharge planner at the hospital notified you that your mother would be ready for discharge tomorrow. The options were for her to go to a skilled nursing facility until she was able to live independently again or go home with you. You manage a department store in addition to being married and having two teenage children. You struggle with the issue of having to send your mother to a skilled nursing facility. Finally, after reviewing your budget and your mother's insurance coverage (Medicare A), you decide you can afford to have a home health aide come into your home to help care for your mother.

1. What are the benefits of having your mother stay with you to receive home health care rather than being sent to a skilled nursing facility?
2. What medical team members might come into the home to provide care for her? Why would their services be needed?
3. What conditions must be met before your mother's Medicare insurance will pay for services rendered?
4. List at least three "do's and don'ts" of documentation that the physical therapist should be aware of when documenting your mother's care.
5. What are three time-management strategies that the home health medical providers could use to help contain your mother's home health costs?

CHECK YOUR RESPONSES

1. Benefits of home care:
    *   Mother will be more comfortable in a home environment.
    *   She will have an increased motivation level and sense of control.
    *   She will be surrounded by people who love her.
    *   Home care is less expensive than an SNF.

2. Medical team members who might provide care and why their services might be needed:
    *   Nursing care: Nursing care might be needed to monitor wound healing, change dressings, as well as monitor her medication and hypertension until she can get into a car to go to the physician's office.
    *   Physical therapy: A physical therapist might come into the home to help increase your mother's range of motion, strength, and balance, assess the safety of the home (ie, area rugs, night lights, steps), evaluate equipment needs (ie, 3-in-1 chair, shower bars, front-wheeled walker, etc). The physical therapist will also monitor your mother's blood pressure and other physical signs and symptoms she may exhibit.
    *   Home health aide: A home health aide might be present to help care for the daily needs of your mother (ie, bathing, dressing, cooking, etc).

3. Conditions that must be met before your mother's care will be covered by Medicare.
    *   The care includes intermittent skilled nursing care, physical therapy, or speech therapy.
    *   The individual must be confined to the home (homebound).
    *   The individual must be under the care of a physician who determines that the individual needs home care and who set up the home care plan.
    *   The home care agency providing the covered services must be certified as a participant in the Medicare program.

4. Do's and don'ts of documentation. The following should be documented:
    *   Reason the patient is homebound
    *   Objective findings of the evaluation and progress made on re-evaluation
    *   Functional goals and timelines
    *   Treatment plan should be related to functional goals
    *   Home program instructions
    *   Safety hazards
    *   Plan for discharge from the first visit

- All conferences with all health care team members (ie, occupational therapy, physical therapy, SLP, nursing, home health aide)

Do not use the following terms:
- Patient is "stabilized" (if not planning to discharge).
- Patient is "doing well" (state what the patient has done to overcome his or her limitation)
- "Maintains" range of motion or strength
- Use arrows or terms such as increase or decrease without including specific objective measures (ie, increase from 20° flexion to 45° flexion)
- "Same" on each visit note

5. Time-management and cost-containment strategies:
   - Schedule mother's visit as well as other patients who live in the same area in a cluster of time. This will prevent wasting driving time.
   - Get clear, concise directions to the house.
   - Mail or fax a home evaluation form to the family to complete prior to the visit.
   - Have suggestions and phone numbers ready of certain medical supply companies that are dependable and will more than likely be able to meet your mother's needs.
   - Be familiar with mother's insurance carrier and the medical equipment it will authorize. This will help avoid reimbursement denial in the future.

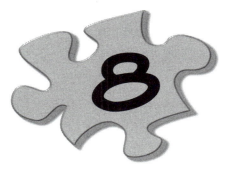

TIME MANAGEMENT TECHNIQUES

Noelle Righter-Freer, MPT

Stanley, a practicing physical therapist of 10 years, prides himself on the quality care he provides at the university medical center. He is known for the quality time and hands-on attention he gives to each one of his patients. However, he has become increasingly frustrated with the concerns of his supervisors to increase his productivity. As the situation currently stands, he feels that 30 minutes is just barely enough to provide his patients quality treatment time. He finds himself constantly behind on his appointments and annoyed by aides who appear to be standing around while he is scrambling from patient to patient. He attributes this to late patient arrivals, nontherapeutic needs of the patients during therapy sessions, pager interruptions, and increased paperwork resulting from "newly imposed managed care red tape." Stanley is experiencing increasing difficulty with devoting full attention to his patients during therapy, as his mind is distracted by numerous details he must tend to before his day is complete. Finding himself working longer days, yet accomplishing less, he confides in his supervisor, stating, "There's no way I can continue my level of quality care within these time crunches. Maybe I'm not cut out to practice physical therapy in this drive-through therapy environment."

Stacey, a practicing therapist of 2 years, also prides herself on the quality care she provides at the university medical center. She works toward improving evaluation efficiency by performing initial necessary screenings in 30 minutes and continuing to evaluate as needed. She works to maximize her treatment sessions to use nontherapeutic time (patient transfers, bathroom visits) thera- peutically, which saves her the frustration of not executing the entire proposed therapeutic exercise regime in an hour. Often, she is able to treat more than three patients in 1 hour by implementing group therapeutic exercise sessions and delegating ancillary treatment responsibilities to aides. Stacey is assertive in discouraging late patient arrivals, interdisciplinary treatment run-overs, and phone call interruptions. She blocks out 1 hour of time at the end of each day and uses "down-time" to complete documentation, order equipment, and return phone calls. Stacey consistently completes her entire patient load and documentation within her scheduled 8-hour day. She is encouraged by her patients' outcomes despite her lack of experience in con- trast to her colleagues. She is presently establishing a mentoring program for her department, as she is grateful for the time her mentor spent sharing her time-saving strategies.

(Ideas for case study generated from Kovacek, P. The productive PT. PT-Magazine of Physical Therapy. 1996;4(4):33-36.)

How is it possible for one therapist to fit everything in while the other is continually frustrated and behind? The major difference between Stanley and Stacey lies in their time management skills.

This chapter addresses *time management*, "...managing ourselves to best use the time we have, to learn to function within the time available, and to achieve satisfactory results."[1] It all boils down to managing yourself, rather than time itself.[2] Time management is an important tool to master to avoid Stanley's predicament—riding on the fast track to burn-out.[3]

Stanley feels that he cannot provide quality treatment without providing 30 minutes of one-on-one time. He feels that his patients are "shorted" if he del- egates too much of the patients' treatment to support personnel. When asked to increase his efficiency, he immediately feels defensive; to him, increased effi- ciency means cutting out valuable treatment time. Stanley might perceive that Stacey has chosen to compromise quality treatment to increase time efficien- cy. Stacey may argue that her patient outcomes are just as good as Stanley's even though she is able to treat more patients per hour. Is her perception real- istic?

Demonstrated above are two different perceptions of "quality" treatment. With the challenges of staff reductions, increased patient loads, and increased time constraints, Stanley, like many therapists, believes productivity is becoming a priority over quality treatment in the face of managed care trends.[4-6] Stacey believes she is in control of the impending pressures to become more productive. She has developed the ability to recognize potential interferences that will set her schedule behind and addresses them before they become a problem. She is able to differentiate what patient treatment is vital for her to address during treatment time and what can be efficaciously delegated to support personnel or taught to the patient and family. She realizes that she is spending less time with her patients, but her outcomes demonstrate that her therapy is effective.

Stacey has realized that excellent training in school is useless if she does not learn how to apply it in an environment with constraints. This is realistic. When adapting to these trends, it is important to keep in mind that quality does not necessarily maintain an inverse relationship with productivity. When time is managed properly, you will find that quality and productivity are mutually attainable.[4-10]

To completely appreciate the positive correlation between these two aspects of treatment, clinicians must look at how they define quality. If quality is defined as "efficient, accountable, and likely to provide the desired outcome,"[1] then it can co-exist with productive treatment. As demonstrated in the above examples, clinicians who are treating with both quality and efficiency find that it is a matter of working smarter not harder.[1,7,10,11]

CHANGE YOUR MINDSET

This is the most important strategy to employ. Time management is more than a list of "how to" strategies; it is a state of mind. However, to change your mindset requires you to know yourself. This means knowing your behaviors, your bad habits, and your self-imposed time management problems that inhibit your ability to have the most effective work day possible. Knowing yourself also requires you to know where you are spending your time. A helpful model, developed by Steven Covey[11] and displayed in Table 8.1, demonstrates four categories (or quadrants) in which most people spend their workday: I. important and urgent, II. important and nonurgent, III. nonimportant and urgent, and IV. Unimportant and nonurgent. Where do you as a physical therapist spend most of your time? Refer to the explanation below to find out where you should be spending most of your time.[11,12]

I. Important, Nonurgent Activities

This is where you as a physical therapist need to be. Within this quadrant,

TABLE 8.1

THE COVEY TIME MANAGEMENT MATRIX

	Urgent	Not urgent
Important	Crises; pressing problems; deadline-driven projects	Prevention, production capability activities; relationship building; recognizing new opportunities; planning; recreation
Not important	Interruptions; some calls; some mail/reports; some meetings; proximate pressing matters; popular activities	Trivia, busy work; some mail; some phone calls; time wasters; pleasant activities

Adapted from Frings CS. Working harder and getting nowhere—no wonder you are stressed! Nursing Administration Quarterly. 1993;18(1):51-56.

you are pro-active rather than reactive. Your emphasis is on important, nonurgent activities, with less problem-oriented management taking place and more goal accomplishment. Time spent working toward your goals increases your satisfaction and decreases your stress. You are able to delegate effectively so that more of your time is spent troubleshooting, counseling, and monitoring progress toward the stated goals.

II. Important, Urgent Activities

Generally, there are three reasons why an individual would be functioning in this quadrant:
1. Patient needs
2. Internal forces (staff, resources, and environment)
3. External forces (the economy, weather, politics, etc)

Patient needs may be urgent but, because they are the nature of physical therapy practice, many of these needs can be anticipated. Additionally, internal forces can be dealt with ahead of time with the use of contingency plans. If external forces can be predicted (ie, economic changes), planning can minimize their impact.

III. Unimportant, Urgent Activities

The unimportant, urgent activities in this quadrant are often not critical to the physical therapist's goals. Their urgency is established by superiors. Examples of these activities include reports that are never read and projects that do not contribute to the organization's mission. Eliminating these activities from your workload may be difficult. Therefore, at the very least, vow to never created urgent, unimportant work for your staff.

IV. Unimportant, Nonurgent Activities

Time spent in this quadrant should be avoided. This quadrant is for nonurgent and unimportant activities. If the activities are not urgent or important, then they are a waste of time.

"IF TIME IS FLYING, WHO'S THE PILOT?"[8]

Constantly think, "What is the best use of my time right now?[5] Is my time being used effectively as well as efficiently?" Putting yourself in the appropriate quadrant may be accomplished by putting some of the following strategies to use:

- Be pro-active, not reactive. You are in control. Learn to anticipate changes imposed by managed care trends and evaluate how you can make your treatment better and more efficient under the imposed restrictions. View them as challenges, not obstacles.[11,13,14]
- Know what is most important in your role as a physical therapist. Lack of clear goals, direction, focus, and ultimately, extended work days occur as a result of not tending to those things most pertinent to your role as a physical therapist. Many therapists are torn between spending enough time with patients and tending to other administrative duties. Commit yourself to spending time in those areas that are most important in terms of your job duties, authority, and responsibility levels.[13,15]
- Be motivated to change your behaviors to better manage your time. This requires commitment, discipline, and desire to change. Avoid discouragement if you don't master time management right away. Set small goals and remember time management is a process that requires time!
- Be creative. As resources are removed, brainstorm for effective alternatives on quality treatment. Creativity can also be used as you fight to retain your resources. You can learn a lot from watching and consulting effective time managers. Ideas can be generated from co-workers, managers in other disciplines, and by taking seminars and reading books that address time management.[9]
- Be flexible. Be prepared to adapt to more challenges. The only consistency in planned schedules is inconsistency.[9]

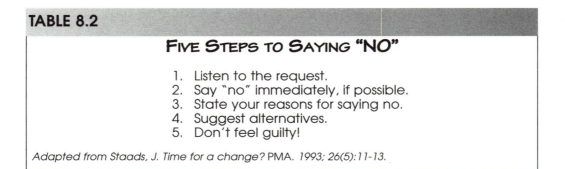

TABLE 8.2

FIVE STEPS TO SAYING "NO"

1. Listen to the request.
2. Say "no" immediately, if possible.
3. State your reasons for saying no.
4. Suggest alternatives.
5. Don't feel guilty!

Adapted from Staads, J. Time for a change? PMA. 1993; 26(5):11-13.

- Be assertive: learn to say "no." This prevents you from cramming too much into your schedule and being less effective at everything. Don't fool yourself into thinking that by saying, "I'll think about it and will get back to you," will buy you time if you really don't intend to commit. Saying "no" even when it hurts becomes less painful when you are direct and honest (Table 8.2).[14,16,17]
- Enforce no-show and late-arrival policies.
- Be assertive with physicians, nurses, and other staff members to complete requests.

As Catherine Deering suggests, ask yourself the following questions when deciding whether or not to refuse a request:[18]

1. If I say yes, will I resent the other person?
2. What will doing this cost me?
3. Does this request conflict with my values?
4. How valuable is my time, and is this request important enough to spend time on?
   - Recognize your limitations. Don't be a perfectionist. Recognize that sometimes it is impossible to accomplish everything.[8] Come to terms with the fact that you cannot be everything to everybody. This will require you to prioritize your values.[15] If you are forced to choose where to allocate your time, leave those duties that do not coincide with these values for last or don't do them at all. Reward yourself for those things you do get done, rather than feel guilty for those things you can't get done.[19]
   - View the patient as a care partner, not a care receiver. This requires the patient to be responsible for participation in his or her own care. If the patient is motivated to maximize his or her time and energy on the home program, you will be freed to pursue other priorities during his or her treatment time.[7]

AVOID THE "TIME WARP"

Keep a Daily Log

It is difficult to modify time-wasting behaviors if you are not aware of where your time is going. You may find your time easier to track if you take a couple of days to jot down on paper what you are doing each hour in a daily log. For example, if you know that a routine patient with a fractured hip should only require 30 minutes of treatment, write down the time when you enter the patient's room and again when you complete the treatment. This will make you aware of the fact that you may be spending extra time in this activity. Next, identify three areas in your log that are consistently and unnecessarily taking up your time. Make it a goal to work on cutting down on time spent in these areas.[20]

Once you have identified your patterns of time-wasting behavior, form a daily log of how you would like to spend your time and stick to it. For instance, make it a goal to spend only 45 minutes on a cervical evaluation. Be realistic and don't make the mistake of allocating too little time for a job that takes longer.[1,14,15]

Now that you've developed a sense for your personal time wasters, there may be more that you are not aware of in the sections below (Table 8.3). Although they appear to be simple and common sense, they are not consistently practiced by experienced clinicians.[7]

Addressing Paperwork

Don't procrastinate. Write down as much as you remember as soon as you can. The longer you wait to record details, the longer it will take to catch up later. Trying to recall all of them will take you twice as long. This principle applies to all administrative aspects of the physical therapist's work day.[1,5,6,18,21]

Paperwork shortcuts and strategies:
- **Use short breaks and down-time.** Always carry blank progress notes with you, so you can record while you are waiting for a patient.
- **Dictate instead of writing, if at all possible.** It will take much less time than writing the same information.
- **Use pre-printed forms and flow sheets for therapeutic exercise and documentation.** Photocopy Medicare forms and fill in only the sections for updated patient progress and a new date. Prior to patient evaluation, have them fill out a pre-printed initial history form while they are in the waiting room. This will cut down on your evaluation time.

TABLE 8.3

DANGER ZONE!
KEY TIME WASTERS

- Procrastination
- Telephone interruptions
- Drop-in visitors
- Administering treatment that does not get to source of the problem
- Crises, "putting out fires"
- Lack of objectives
- Lack of deadlines
- Unrealistic time estimates
- Cluttered desk
- Personal disorganization
- Ineffective delegation, attempting too much
- Gripes, complaints, morale situations
- Confused responsibilities
- Inability to say no

- Leaving tasks unfinished
- Lack of self-discipline
- Losing things
- Conflicting instructions
- Not doing tasks correctly
- Lack of a checklist
- Failure to listen
- Doing it yourself
- Daydreaming/ lack of concentration
- Excessive socializing/ excessive small talk with patients
- "Standing by" for patient preparation for treatment or for staff member discussions
- Lack of clear communication

Adapted from Frings CS. Effective time management. Medical Laboratory Observer. *1988; 20(7):43-45; and Stewart N.* The Effective Woman Manager. *New York: John Wiley and Sons; 1981.*

- **Keep notes clear yet concise.** Use better wording and abbreviations to shorten your sentences.
- **Never handle a piece of paper more than once.** Take action, address it, discard it, pass it on, or file it away.
- **Avoid distractions.** Find a time of day that you know will have limited interruptions. If you are interrupted, politely, but firmly, enforce a "do not disturb" policy. Stopping and starting up again are big time wasters. If you do need to stop during paperwork, stop in mid-sentence. This will serve as a "memory trigger" to ease your flow back into writing when you are able to resume.[22]

Be Aware of Miscellaneous Time Wasters

- **Carry a pager.** This will cut down on unnecessary trips to check messages or waiting on communication.
- **Cut down on meetings.** These are big time-wasters. Try to accomplish as much as possible while everyone is there. If you are conducting the meeting, have a pre-printed agenda and stick to it. It is helpful to conduct "meetings in hallways," that is, a brief, informal meeting involving two to four people to arrive at a consensus or share information.[14]

- **Avoid ancillary tasks.** You are paid $20 (or more) an hour to exercise your unique skills and expertise. Do so only if you have true down-time.
- **Delegate.** Support personnel are there to assist you in maximizing patient treatment quality and efficiency.
- **Recognize the worth of others' time.** Confining your treatment to scheduled times will encourage other staff members to respect your time slots as well.[4]

TOOLS TO CREATE TIME

With a day jam-packed with miscellaneous information, important details can get lost in the shuffle. It is vital that you have a systematic way of keeping track of what you are supposed to do. You may want to try the following suggestions.[5]

- **"To-do" lists.** Make a list of priorities that need to be addressed before your day is over.
- **Calendar/day planner.** Schedule all that needs to be accomplished and allow realistic time to get it done.
- **Tickler file.** This file is to remain in front of your patient file box. This is a file that should be organized according to months. It can consist of reminders for patients that need to be brought to your attention in following visits. It also can consist of reminders (ie, equipment ordering, Medicare deadlines) that need to be brought to your attention weeks and months down the road.
- **Hot file.** As the name sounds, this file is urgent. Place matters here that need to be taken care of in 1 to 2 days.
- **Color coding.** Filing systems can be color coded for clarity. Whatever system you choose to use or invent, make sure all of your materials and resources are kept in one place.

BLOCK OUT!

Documentation, phone calls, junk mail, and notes to doctors can add a minimum of 2 hours to your day or can invade your weekend if they are not handled efficiently. Ironically, managing time requires you to put "time" into it. You may find it useful to reduce 10 patients' treatment times by 5 minutes to create an extra hour at the end of the day to address miscellaneous tasks. Be consistent and hold yourself accountable to the following routine.

Block Out Time Once an Hour

- **Schedule paperwork time.** Save 5 minutes at the end of each treatment session to record patient progress. Don't procrastinate! Record evaluative data and progress notes as soon as possible.
- **Organize equipment.** Carry all necessary items on your person. Be aware of patients' needs for therapy (ie, walker, hand dynamometer). This way, you can avoid needless trips backtracking to your office.
- **Set up equipment** before a patient comes into an outpatient setting. Arrange high-usage equipment in an accessible, convenient location to avoid wasted time searching for it.
- **In the acute setting,** take down equipment such as continuous passive motion units and IV poles; adjust bed rails as you are talking to patients or taking a subjective history.
- **Schedule the next visit.** Give patients options for scheduling their next visit while they are in their treatment rooms dressing. This will give them time to organize their own schedules by the time they arrive at the scheduling desk. If you have the luxury of employing front office personnel, make sure these tasks are delegated to them.
- **Prioritize patient outcomes.** Remind yourself of the patient's best interests and outcomes during each treatment. After a quick assessment, prioritize the most important goals for the patient within the imposed time constraints.
- **Avoid "treating tangents"** and getting side-tracked by the patient's secondary problems. Avoid the urge to follow your personal interests or goals that are not shared by the patient.[6,7]

Block Out Time Once a Day

- **Focus on goals.** Keep focused on your personal goals throughout the day. Keep the big picture of your primary role as a therapist and take steps toward that goal. This may require you to post a "to-do" list. If at all possible, complete the cycle of the task you have begun before starting a new one.
- **Review your schedule.** Check your daily planner and patient schedule so you can anticipate what lies ahead. Make changes and block out a personal time for housekeeping and errands. This ensures that no patients are scheduled, so you can be sure to avoid interruptions. Organize for the following day the night before.[14]
- **Check your hot file.** This file is intended for urgent matters that cannot afford to be put off more than 1 or 2 days.
- **Phone calls.** Set aside time to make all phone calls at once. Log your messages and phone calls, and try to keep them in one place.

- **Replenish blank progress note sheets.** Make a pile of all outpatient progress sheets at the beginning of each day to eliminate unnecessary trips back and forth to the office. Always put these back as well!
- **Monitor potential problems.** Check in with support personnel in the morning and/or afternoon for questions or to handle emergency situations. It is your responsibility to troubleshoot potential problems with delegation. Don't take it for granted that they will come to you.

Block Out Time Once a Week

- **Review current charts.** Check charts weekly. This will ensure that charts are caught up and not missing any details, such as cosignatures, case conferences, or progress notes.
- **Review next week's schedule.** Check your calendar and patient schedule. Be prepared for the events coming up in your next week. Update all events, meetings, or patient documentation that has not yet been recorded. Prepare staff if they are involved in any arrangement that concerns you.
- **Check tickler file.** Check this file to see if there is anything you overlooked. If there is anything missing, update it. Address the patient reminders that need attention right away!
- **Catch up!** If for some unavoidable reason you have been forced to put off paperwork, catch up on it at the end of the week. Try not to let the next week begin with this pile hanging over your head.[5]

WHY BOTHER?
I DON'T HAVE TIME TO MANAGE MY TIME!

The benefits that you reap from investing time and effort into time management will be worthwhile. It begins first by placing yourself into a time management mindset. Establishing an aggressive attitude toward time management will make you more effective in avoiding the "time warp" in combating miscellaneous time wasters, addressing paperwork, putting time management tools to use, and "blocking out" time hourly, daily, and weekly.

These time savers will allow you more freedom for tasks that require your professional skills and expertise. You will find time to reflect and be creative, set goals, organize, widen your referral base, plan inservices, develop programs, expand your education, as well as spend more time working with patients of higher complexities.

When you manage your time efficiently, your department will run more smoothly if you are busy or are on vacation. Support personnel will benefit from their increased time with patients and will learn to adapt to increased responsibilities. They will have a chance to perfect their skills, as well as improve their confidence and motivation. A change of atmosphere will occur not only when you are there, but also when you are away.[24]

The benefits of time management are endless. You will be more effective at combating burn-out as you find more time for rest, relaxation, and those loved ones most important to you.[14] Following these strategies will keep the physical therapy profession at the forefront, making us more effective professionals and increasing referral access, as we will be able to reach more of the population and reap more satisfaction while doing it.[25]

REFERENCES

1. Barros A. Time management: learn to work smarter, not harder. *Medical Laboratory Observer.* 1983; 15(8):106-111.
2. Byrd EK. Time management in a rehabilitation setting. *Journal of Rehabilitation.* 1982: 48:47-50.
3. Curtis KA, Martin T. Perceptions of acute care physical therapy practice; issues for physical therapist preparation. *Phys Ther,* 1993;73(9):581-597.
4. Knortz K. Increasing productivity in the acute care setting. *Physical Therapy Forum.* 1990;9(46):2-5.
5. Curtis K. *Ideas for Managing Unmanageable Caseloads.* Los Angeles: Health Directions; 1986.
6. Salo B. Ten tips for paperwork management. *Physical Therapy Forum.* 1991; 11:140.
7. Personal communication. Bullock, Kathy, Director of Older Adult Services, St. Mary's Medical Center, Long Beach, Calif, July 15, 1996.
8. Tyner T. California State University Fresno. Course in Introduction to Supervision in Physical Therapy Services, lecture notes, September 18, 1995.
9. Personal communication. Boyles-Haubursin, Dawan, Director of Clinical Services, San Joaquin Valley Rehabilitation Hospital. Fresno, Calif, July 19, 1996.
10. Kovacek P. The productive PT. *PT-Magazine of Physical Therapy.* 1996;4(4):33-35.
11. Frings CS. Working harder and getting nowhere—no wonder you are stressed! *Nursing Administration Quarterly.* 1993;18(1):55-56.
12. Personal communication. McCubbin, Annette, California State University, Fresno. Seminar in Health Care Issues I, May 5, 1997.
13. Time management: knowledge for practice. *Nursing Times.* 1994;90(27):1-4.
14. McCormack MH. *What They Don't Teach You at Harvard Business School: Notes from a Street Smart Executive.* New York: Bantam Books; 1988.
15. Schuler RS. Managing stress means managing time. *Personnel Journal.* 1979; 58(12):851-854.
16. Staads J. Time for a change? *PMA.* 1993; 26(5):11-13.
17. Laver R. Taking charge of time. *Maclean's.* 1997;110(4):53.
18. Deering CG. Learning to say no: Simple steps you can take to protect yourself from over committing your time and energy. *Am J Nurs.* 1996;96(4):62-64.

19. Rondeau KV. Procrastination means lost productivity. *Canadian Journal of Medical Technology.* 1993;55(2):74-76.

20. Frings CS. Effective time management. *Medical Laboratory Observer.* 1988; 20(7):43-45.

21. Carter R. Write it now, or never! *Nurse Author and Editor.* 1996:6(2):3-4,7.

22. Winston S. *The Organized Executive: New Ways to Manage Time, Paper, People, and the Electronic Office.* New York: W.W. Norton and Co., Inc.; 1994.

23. Stewart N. *The Effective Woman Manager.* New York: John Wiley and Sons; 1981.

24. Raudsepp E, Januz L. Do you delegate, or do it yourself? *Executive.* 1989:16-19.

25. Macan TH. Time management: test of a process model. *J Appl Psychol.* 1994; 79(3):381-391.

26. Personal communication, group interview. Julie Hall, Kyndra Gean, and Cheri Parks, California State University, Fresno. September 15, 1996.

TEST YOUR SKILLS

You are responsible for the care of all patients in the following list. After arranging your patient agenda for the day, you check your "In-Box," which consists of the following stack of paperwork. As the day progresses, you encounter the tertiary list of Murphy's Law challenges. You must rearrange your schedule to accommodate the following inconveniences. Please fit all of the necessary tasks and treatments into your schedule book between 8:00 am to 5:00 pm. Use support personnel consisting of two aides and a physical therapist assistant (PTA). Keep in mind that you are only paid for 8 hours a day.[26]

	Your schedule	PTA	Physical therapy aide #1	Physical therapy aide #2
8:00 am				
8:30 am				
9:00 am				
9:30 am				
10:00 am				
10:30 am				
11:00 am				
11:30 am				
12:00 pm				
12:30 pm				
1:00 pm				
1:30 pm				
2:00 pm				
2:30 pm				
3:00 pm				
3:30 pm				
4:00 pm				
4:30 pm				

Physical therapy patients to be seen:
- 70 y.o. patient with total knee replacement evaluated yesterday, need to order a walker
- 30 y.o. patient with total knee replacement, third follow-up treatment
- 75 y.o. patient with vestibular/balance disorder for gait training
- 13 y.o. patient with gunshot wound to brachial plexus evaluated yesterday
- 22 y.o. patient with closed head injury 10 days post-general ROM
- Evaluation 68 y.o. patient with hip ORIF 1 day postop
- Evaluation patient with right hemiplegia/post-CVA
- 60 y.o. patient with hip ORIF crutch training, needs to order home commode

- 14 y.o. patient with femur fracture, dislocated shoulder 5 days post-MVA, crutch training
- 7 y.o. patient with muscular dystrophy, 5 days postop, Achilles tendon release, ROM
- 38 y.o. patient with MVA cervical strain, pubic rami hairline fracture, 10 days post-injury, gait training
- Evaluation 45 y.o. patient with myocardial infarction 3 days post-episode

Paper work/housekeeping:
- Update three Medicare forms, update due tomorrow
- Call physician for weight-bearing status on patient with hip ORIF
- Write up two new evaluations that were performed yesterday
- Call for authorization from two private insurers
- Former cardiac patient with chest pains called for modification of home program.
- Family friend called for advice for daughter, as she "hurt her knee" playing basketball
- Call physician for referral to extend treatment, as he has not returned the last three phone calls
- Grandma's birthday gift must be mailed today to arrive on time
- You are conducting a staff organizational meeting scheduled over your lunch hour

Murphy's Law:
- Your son's principal calls you to pick him up, as he was caught "smoking in the boy's room"
- 7 y.o. patient with muscular dystrophy takes 30 minutes, occupied with bathroom activities
- 60 y.o. patient with hip ORIF refuses treatment
- One aide goes home sick at 1:00 pm
- PTA expresses frustration with the "way he has been treated" and requests a personal conference

CHECK YOUR RESPONSES

First, consider the urgency and importance of each task on the list. What must you do yourself? What can you delegate to others? What can you put off until tomorrow or the following day?

Be sure to create a plan that meets legal and ethical guidelines and support personnel supervisory requirements in your state.

Have you allowed time for documentation, time for telephone calls, time for communication with other members of the team?

What items are most highly prioritized on your "to do" list?

You may want to come back and review your responses after reading Chapter 9. Caseload management and time management are related skills. You may gain additional ideas that will change your plan.

Compare your responses with those of your colleagues and discuss the rationale for your decisions.

CASELOAD MANAGEMENT AND DELEGATION

Noelle Righter-Freer, MPT

*J*anice Williams is the senior physical therapist in charge of directing the county medical center's physical therapy department. She is diligent in sticking to her plan of conducting weekly staff meetings to keep the department running smoothly. This Monday morning, the staff begins to venture off the agenda as the conversation begins to turn into a venting session. Concerns expressed sound something like this:

Sal Rodriguez, RPT: I have been practicing at this facility for 24 years, and I have never seen patients shipped in and shipped out so quickly as I have this past year. I mean, they sent an 80-year-old woman with a fractured hip home in 1 week! So much for carrying out my treatment plan.

Dana Thomas, MPT: You think that is bad? Yesterday I had to treat three patients with fractured hips in 1 hour. That's been about the norm lately; I have no time to fit in everything I want to do with them.

Iman Farage, PT aide: No wonder you have been filling my schedule so full, Dana. I have been working with 14 of your patients per day. To be honest, even though I've been here for 7 years, I don't feel confident performing some of the treatments you ask me to.

Kelly Davidson, PTA: When are we going to hire another PT? Patients are complaining that they never have the same person treat them. I probably hear about it most because I'm part-time and hardly ever see the same patient twice. It's very hard for me to provide them with continuity of care with my assigned patient load.

Dana: I'm sorry, but it's been really difficult for me to stand over you every minute of the day with all of the directions that I'm being pulled.

Sal: You don't have to tell me about "difficult." I had to discharge someone the other day before I even had the chance to instruct his family on how to assist him. That reminds me, I wanted to discuss her case in more detail with Dr. Cunningham. I rarely have time to discuss anything with any doctors anymore.

Janice: I understand all of your concerns. I did 30 evaluations myself last week. We're really short of help right now because of the staff turnover rate. But we've all got to work together to take control of this situation. There is a waiting list of referrals we've got to cut down. We've lost a lot of good staff members lately, and I don't want to lose any of you.

All of the concerns expressed above have one thing in common: difficulty with caseload management. *Caseload management* "requires the ability to manage a number of clients within a given amount of time and provide optimum service."[1] Conversations similar to this are becoming increasingly common in clinical settings everywhere. How would you respond to these concerns if you were the director?

As a physical therapist juggling numerous responsibilities within a heavy caseload, it is important to abide by appropriate time- and cost-efficient strategies within ethical and legal guidelines. The following chapter provides solutions addressing many caseload dilemmas such as these. Although they appear to be simple common sense, they are not consistently practiced by experienced clinicians.[2,3]

SHARPEN YOUR SKILLS

Before you evaluate your patient, you must first evaluate yourself. You may find that you need to brush up, fine tune, or even relearn skills that indirectly can have a major impact on condensing your caseload.[4]

- **Sharpen your diagnostic skills.** With all of the continuing education available, it can be an overwhelming choice deciding on where and when to spend your weekends and money learning to specialize on what skills. In light of maximizing visits with your patients, there is nothing more valuable than being able to determine the specificity of their primary problem. Once this is established, address this problem in a treatment approach that will most quickly and effectively regain their function. Otherwise, you will waste valuable treatment time and visits "chasing your tail" trying to eliminate deceptive symptoms.[4] For instance, being able to differentiate a rotator cuff impingement from bursitis will help you to address the problem more efficiently, enabling a faster return of function.

- **Sharpen your interpersonal communication skills.** When dealing with difficult or demanding patients, be aware of what motivates and positively encourages them. This will save you and the patient from spending treatment time discussing, convincing, and coaxing.

- **Sharpen your teaching skills.** Change your treatment approach to be more educational. Teach patients, their families, and caregivers tasks to work on at home. Have them demonstrate a thorough understanding of what they have learned, so you can rest assured that they are performing tasks correctly and safely without your supervision. Patients will be guided to take a more active role in their own healing process. This will also allow you to focus on priorities during the treatment session that require your unique expertise.[3]

- **Sharpen your prevention skills.** Approach all your patient treatments with prevention in the back of your mind. This will teach your patients to assume responsibility to avoid aggravating or recreating the same lesion and returning down the road to repeat the same therapy. It will also reduce incidences of "starting from square one" between visits or having to address new secondary problems in addition to the patient's original diagnosis.[2,4]

- **Sharpen your referral skills.** Last but not least, know when to refer. This requires you to recognize your limitations. A good rule of thumb to follow: If your patient does not show improvement by three sessions, re-evaluate your approach. You may need to involve a colleague, seek consultation from your mentor, refer your patient to someone with more experience or specialized education, or, ultimately return your patient to see his or her physician.[4]

DON'T GET CAUGHT SLEEPING!

The changing environment requires you to stay on your toes, constantly aware of what you are doing not only when you are in the room with your patient, but also before he or she arrives and after he or she leaves. It will be helpful to keep a mental checklist that will organize you and help to save time in three stages: (1) before patient treatment, (2) during patient treatment, and (3) after patient treatment. The following strategies may be used in the acute or outpatient rehabilitation setting, or both (unless specified); so use your creativity to apply them to any situation.

Before Patient Treatment

- **Be prepared.** Ensuring that your caseload is handled smoothly requires preparation before the patient even enters the treatment area. Be prepared for new orders for inpatients, as well as new evaluations for outpatients. Be aware of how much time it takes to evaluate a patient with a total knee replacement versus a patient with an above-knee amputation, and allow for time accordingly. If you have early access to your schedule, consult references before the patient arrives so that you can be mentally prepared if it is a diagnosis with which you are not familiar.[5]

- **Prioritize, prioritize, prioritize!** Set goals and priorities for each patient, and focus on those. For example, in acute care settings, patients may have as few as two to three visits before discharge. In these situations, you have no choice but to focus on safety and function. For outpatient settings, work-hardening skills may be most important to address for a patient anxious to return to work.[5]

- **Plan for discharge.** Be aware of the discharge course before treatment. If you don't know the next level of care your patient is headed for, how can you be effective in getting him or her there? This information will also help you direct the course of treatment. For example, if the patient is headed for home discharge, then focus on functional home activities in therapy.[1,6]

- **Know the limitations of the patient's coverage.** Familiarize yourself with the patient's reimbursement method prior to treatment. Knowing what his or her insurance will not cover and the number of authorized visits may change your course of treatment.[2]

- **Do your own scheduling.** If possible, schedule your own patients. If this is not realistic, have someone who is aware of your patient needs do so. For instance, if you have to schedule another patient at the same time as a more involved cerebrovascular accident (CVA) patient, schedule a patient who is more independent in the gym, requiring minimal supervision.[4]

- **Dove-tail**. This is an effective strategy for treating more than one patient at once. While one patient is receiving a passive modality, you can be working one-on-one with the other. If you know one patient needs to be re-evaluated for discharge, schedule him or her with a patient who needs to receive heat for the first 20 minutes of treatment. By the time you are finished with the re-evaluation, both patients may be ready for you to simultaneously supervise them in the gym.[7]
- **Stagger patient arrival times.** Staggering patient start times every 15 to 20 minutes allows you time to prepare modality and equipment or even review the patient's chart prior to his or her arrival. This will prevent one patient from waiting for you while you are setting up for another.[7]
- **Co-treat.** You can accomplish more with the help of an occupational therapist (OT) or other staff member. While you are working on a neurological patient's trunk stability in sitting, the OT can be addressing fine motor movements with upper extremities. This will teach the patient to coordinate upper extremity work in a variety of positions, as well as save the patient an extra hour of therapy.[2]
- **Co-evaluate.** If possible, arrange a program in which you are able to coordinate the same evaluation time with the physician, OT, nurse, and/or speech pathologist. This will eliminate repetitions of tests and history questions. It is a great way to exchange information with other disciplines and learn more about your patient. It also constitutes a greater team effort upon which to coordinate treatment with the other disciplines. This will allow you to gather baseline information and follow up with more details in following visits.[2]
- **Assess progress and modify treatment.** Reassess your patients before treating them. You can avoid wasting time on treatments or modalities that they may no longer need. To avoid repetition throughout evaluation, learn to prioritize specific evaluation tests to determine the patient's primary problem. You can use the time when the patient is receiving a modality to gather more subjective information.[7]
- **Involve others in physical therapy goals.** Inform other disciplines of your physical therapy goals when sharing patients. If your goals are reinforced in the patient's other therapy sessions, you can spend time on other priorities in your following physical therapy sessions. Weekly team conference meetings are a good way to accomplish this task.[6,7]

Before patient treatment in the acute setting

- **Use a schedule board.** Coordinate your schedule with other therapy disciplines and post them on a schedule board. This will avoid confusion between you and other staff members. This will also eliminate double scheduling of the same patient or double scheduling of the same equipment.[7]
- **Be aware of other staff members' schedules**. It is helpful to check with nurs-

ing staff members at the beginning of the day. You may be able to find out patient bathing schedules, to let them know when your patients need to be pre-medicated before therapy, or to coordinate dressing schedules and bedding changes with nursing assistants or aides. This will allow you to work together with nursing assistants or aides if you need assistance for bed mobility or transfers. Nurses may have their own schedule board.

Coordinating with discharge planners in the morning will also make your day run more smoothly. Finding out which patients will be discharged during the day will alert you to treat those patients first or coordinate final family training, equipment issues, or car transfers without having to interrupt treatment with another patient. You can also eliminate time wasted reviewing a chart or searching for a patient who is no longer there.

- **Check the surgery schedule.** Familiarize yourself with the surgery schedule, anticipating new patients who require your immediate attention. If these patients are blocked in your schedule, you will not be faced with squeezing them in when it is time to go home.[7]
- **Prepare patients for treatment.** Verbally prepare inpatients to anticipate treatment. This will enable them to be ready at treatment time both physically and mentally. Be aware of the times during the day when your patients function at their peak performances. For example, some patients function better in the morning when they are not as tired.[7]

During Patient Treatment

- **Plan treatment time and tasks.** Set a timer to remind you when your patients are scheduled to finish modality treatments. Schedule them so that you are not in the middle of another treatment when they require your attention. If you must divert your attention, give them an independent task to do until you're available (ie, stretch, relaxation exercises).[7]
- **Group patients with similar needs.** Use group therapy whenever possible. Schedule and work patients together who are performing the same therapeutic exercises. If two patients need crutch training, train them together. One can watch and rest while the other is practicing. Hearing the directions repeated again will reinforce proper performance, and the patients can gather confidence while watching each other perform. This creates a positive environment for the patients to support each other.[7]
- **Use classes.** Grouping your patients into "back classes" or other ergonomic classes will offer the same information to several patients at once.[7]
- **Use treatment guidelines.** Use critical pathways and protocols as guidelines. Of course, you want to exercise your own clinical decision-making skills to be

creative and flexible, but you don't want to reinvent the wheel. Relying on prior outcome studies and the experience and organization of others will save you time. You can improvise along the way.[2]

- **Use every minute.** Make maximum use of passive modality time. Whether the patient is receiving heat, ice, or electrical stimulation, this time can be used to gather subjective data, review instructions, stretch, or perform isometric contractions.[7] In the acute setting, remove and arrange patient equipment (continuous passive motion machines, IV poles, compression pumps, adjust beds) while you are talking to the patient and gathering subjective data.

- **Keep the patient focused.** Learn to tactfully and politely keep patients focused on treatment. Although it is important to develop rapport and engage in conversation with patients, take care not to let this take priority over treatment. This requires exercising assertiveness with a smile, using a phrase like, "OK, only five more repetitions to go!" Often, it only takes a tactile cue to remind them to continue with the next set of exercises.

- **Use rest time to exercise other muscles.** Use rest time between sets to exercise a different muscle group. Alternating upper extremity exercises with lower extremity exercises allows the patient to rest while still continuing his or her treatment. You may also alternate opposing extremities or agonist/antagonist groups.[7]

After Patient Treatment

- **Update documentation.** Don't forget to schedule time during the patient's allotted treatment time to do required documentation (and charge for it). With every patient you treat after this patient, it will take longer to recall details that you need to record.[3] Refer to your time management skills (see Chapter 8 for tips on quicker documentation).

- **Manage the case.** Keep in mind all of the factors other than "hands-on treatment" that go into patient care, and allow time to take care of these details. This may involve communication with other team members, equipment ordering, or making outside referrals.

- **Plan ahead.** Do what it takes to prepare for the patient's next treatment session while he or she is fresh on your mind. It is helpful to jot down ideas that you plan to add to his or her treatment next time or information that you will need to assess under "plan" on his or her chart.

   Begin planning for the patient's discharge immediately, no matter what stage of recovery the patient is in. Plan your goals with his or her discharge date and destination in mind. This way you will be sure to address the most important interventions first before the patient departs from your care. Planning ahead will prevent being caught off guard if the patient is discharged early.

- **Use your time management skills.** Don't procrastinate, do it now! Procrastination only makes the job take longer.[6] Set up systematic ways of handling routine tasks and then use the system.

DELEGATION

Delegation is key to managing an "unmanageable" caseload. It has been defined as "the allocation of tasks from the position holder with responsibility for achieving objectives to a subordinate who has been given the authority to carry out the task and who reports to the position holder."[8] Maximum caseload efficiency can be achieved if therapists avoid the mistakes of over-protecting their cases or taking this responsibility too lightly.

- **Use of support personnel.** Ask yourself, "Are my services worth their cost or could someone else be doing this?"[4] If someone else can, make sure those tasks are delegated effectively. Support personnel, aides, and PTAs are there to help you improve the quality of care that you provide.

  Once properly oriented and trained, interns can also help manage caseloads. Many therapists may feel they don't have time to take a student. On the contrary, the time that you invest in him or her will be well worth the payback of extra productivity as he or she gains independence.[9] You can't afford to abide by the cliché, "If you want something done right, do it yourself."[8,10-12]

- **Know the staff's strengths and weaknesses.** Know your staff's strengths and weaknesses, and assign tasks that complement them. Give complex tasks to more experienced personnel. Be familiar with the educational background and curriculum of employees such as athletic trainers and exercise physiologists. Take time to address staff weaknesses safely and with proper supervision.[13,14]

- **Follow ethical and legal guidelines.**
  Effective delegation will require you to be aware of limitations! Make sure you are familiar with legal, ethical, and facility guidelines (see Appendix 3, APTA *Standards of Practice*, for a more complete list of ethical and legal guidelines).

Physical Therapy Aides May Not:

- perform direct physical therapy services to patients without the continuous on-site supervision of the physical therapist or PTA (note: In California, the PTA may not supervise the physical therapy aide)
- perform any duties without the discretion and permission of the physical therapist

Physical Therapy Aides May:

- perform procedures and related tasks that have been selected and delegated by the supervising physical therapist
- assist in patient treatment preparation
- assemble/disassemble equipment and perform operational activities, mainte-nance, and transportation
- assist in patient activities under the direction and direct supervision of a physical therapist

Physical Therapist Assistants May Not:

- treat patients if the physical therapist is not accessible by telecommunication
- perform an initial visit for evaluation
- treat patients without a supervisory visit from the physical therapist at least once a month
- re-evaluate a patient response to a change in medical status, change the treatment plan, or plan a discharge without a supervisory visit from a physical therapist

Physical Therapist Assistants May:

- perform physical therapy procedures and related tasks that have been selected and delegated by the supervising physical therapist
- carry out routine operational functions
- supervise the physical therapy aide (not in California; check the State Practice Act for other states)
- document treatment progress
- modify specific treatment procedures in accordance with changes in patient sta-tus within the scope of the established treatment plan

Only a Physical Therapist May:

- interpret referrals and perform evaluations, identify problems, and diagnosis for physical therapy
- develop or modify a plan of care based on the evaluation
- determine which tasks require the expertise of a physical therapist
- delegate and instruct support personnel in services to be rendered, including precautions, special problems, or contraindicated procedures
- conduct timely review of treatment documentation, re-evaluation, and revision of plan
- establish the discharge plan and perform/document a discharge evaluation

Who is responsible?

If you don't remember anything in the above guidelines, remember that the physical therapist is ultimately responsible and liable. In the eyes of the law, you have no one to blame but yourself if a delegated task causes harm to a patient. It is your reputation and license at stake.[11,13]

KEYS TO EFFECTIVE DELEGATION

Communicate Effectively

Everyone involved (patient, staff, and physical therapist) must agree on what job is being delegated. This will prevent frustrations of uncompleted tasks. Find out your support staff's opinion of their roles and understanding of legal guidelines. You may find that their perceptions of their roles differ from yours. This is where your conflict resolution and listening skills will come in handy to improve professional communication and job satisfaction. Reviewing job descriptions with employees annually (yours and theirs) will help to cut down on conflicting perceptions.[13-15]

Train Support Personnel

If you don't have confidence in your staff to delegate, take time to train them. This will save you much more time in the long run.[15] Drawing on information from ethical, legal, and workplace guidelines, decide what is absolutely essential for support personnel to know when working with patients (Table 9.1). Teach them this baseline knowledge and watch their performance in orientation sessions, quarterly inservices, and with one-on-one supervising, if necessary.[10,13]

Teach staff critical thinking skills. This will cut down on questions and interruptions that can be solved with common sense or on-the-job training.[15] You may find staff members will appreciate the opportunity to learn and grow.[16]

Empower Staff to Complete the Task

Don't forget to delegate authority along with responsibility. Frustration will set in if your support personnel are asked to carry out a task, but are unable to carry it out when other staff members don't recognize their authority. Be aware of hospital/workplace policies and don't assign tasks to personnel outside these guidelines.[13,15]

> ### TABLE 9.1
>
> ## Skills for Physical Therapist Support Personnel
>
> **Important baseline skills for physical therapist support personnel:**
> **Basic care**
> - Understanding hospital standards, policies, and procedures
> - Transfers and body mechanics
> - Basic life support
> - Documenting care measures listed above
> - Basic safety issues and infection control
>
> **Communication**
> - Introducing oneself to a patient and his or her family
> - Listening to supervisors and patients
> - Resolving conflicts between oneself and co-workers or patients
> - Giving and receiving feedback
>
> **Decision-making**
> - Prioritizing tasks
> - Deciding what to report to the physical therapist and/or registered nurse
> - Patient rights
> - Handling complaints from patients and families
>
> **Critical thinking**
> - Identifying risks to patients
> - Appropriately reporting a problem quickly to the physical therapist or registered nurse
>
> *Adapted with permission from Parkman CA. Delegation: Are you doing it right? Am J Nurs. 1996;96(9):42-48.*

Make Performance Matter

Always be available to provide feedback. Make sure tasks are completed safely and correctly. Provide constructive criticism when they are not done correctly.[6,16]

Trust Your Intuition

Assume nothing! Ask questions and listen effectively! Many times, support personnel are reluctant to express insecurities or weaknesses involving task performance. This may require you to exercise intuition and attentiveness to discover their skill level.[13,15]

Know Your Patients' Needs

Be aware of special patient needs, such as assistance levels, if they require co-treatment or prefer to be treated by a caregiver of a certain gender. Know which patients require a physical therapist's expertise and skill. Obviously, this type of patient is not appropriate to delegate. Do your best to maintain continuity of care, and assign patients to the same staff member for each treatment.

Monitor Progress and Follow-up

Monitor the patient's progress and treatment response with support personnel. Follow up on inefficiencies, delays, and vague verbal feedback concerning the patient's treatment response. Always check to review how treatment went or to address any questions. It is the physical therapist's responsibility to ensure that the patient's progress is monitored and to address problems.[15,16]

Recognize and Reward Performance

1. Acknowledge good performance. Ask staff for input and problem solving. Communicate to them that you value their opinions.
2. Give feedback and make expectations known, but don't rush in and take over. Acknowledgment of good performance must be more frequent than correction of inadequate performance.
3. Be reasonable about expectations. Demanding perfection will only cause frustration.
4. Be willing to admit that support personnel may be able to do a job as well as or even better than you! Often, patients will relate to and feel more comfortable with certain members of your support staff. Be aware that certain personalities will work better together to maximize patient motivation.[15]

Be Sensitive to Staff Morale

Don't abuse support personnel. Be sensitive to their stress levels and personal schedules. Ask for their suggestions to make the work environment more enjoyable. Split up unpleasant tasks between personnel. It will be noticeable how much more smoothly the setting will run when staff morale is high.[13,15]

Motivate Your Staff

Convey to them that you believe their task is important. If your attitude demonstrates that a task is menial or unpleasant, staff members may, in turn, be less motivated to perform it with effort and enthusiasm.[15]

CHECK YOUR OWN CASELOAD MANAGEMENT SKILLS

Glancing back through the chapter, you now should be able to recognize suggestions that would help Janice Williams respond to the complaints of her staff members in the opening discussion.

Certainly, the staff physical therapists at the county medical center could benefit from evaluating and sharpening their own skills, brushing up on ethical legal guidelines for delegation, and practicing keys to effective delegation. All staff members could benefit from taking advantage of time before, during, and after patient treatment.

Can you locate caseload management weaknesses in your workplace? Just like time management, being an effective caseload manager is a process that does not happen overnight. However, a commitment to effective case management is essential to personal job satisfaction.[3,17]

REFERENCES

1. Anglin LT. Caseload management. A model for agencies and staff nurses. *Home Healthcare Nurse.* 1992;10(3):26-31.
2. Bullock, Kathy, Director of Older Adult Services, St. Mary's Medical Center. Personal interview, Long Beach, Calif, July 15, 1996.
3. Curtis KA, Martin T. Perceptions of acute care physical therapy practice; issues for physical therapist preparation. *Phys Ther.* 1993;73(9):581-597.
4. Ghandour Y, Doriglas A. Lead Physical Therapist and Senior Physical Therapist at Sharp Reese-Stealy Medical Center. Personal interviews, San Diego, Calif, July 22, 1996.
5. Hansten RI, Washburn MJ. Knowing how to delegate. *Am J Nurs.* 1995;95(7):16H-16L.
6. Curtis K. *Ideas for Managing Unmanageable Caseloads.* Los Angeles: Health Directions. 1986.
7. Knortz K. Increasing productivity in the acute care setting. *Physical Therapy Forum.* 1990;9(46):2-5, 6.
8. Ladyshewsky RK. Enhancing service productivity in acute care inpatient settings using a collaborative clinical education model. *Phys Ther.* 1995;75(6):503-510.
9. Robinson AJ, DePalma MT, McCall M. Physical therapist assistants' perceptions of the documented roles of the physical therapist assistant. *Phys Ther.* 1995;75(12):1054-1066.
10. Saunders L. The role of physiotherapy helpers in out-patient physiotherapy services. *Physiotherapy.* 1995;81(7):384-392.
11. Lang C. A survey of how community physiotherapists use their time. *Physiotherapy.* 1996;82(4):222-226.
12. Kovacek P. The productive PT. *PT-Magazine of Physical Therapy.* 1996;4(4):33-35.
13. Parkman CA. Delegation: Are you doing it right? *Am J Nurs.* 1996;96(9):43-47.
14. Bella JM. On decision making. *Phys Ther.* 1996;76(11):1232-1240.
15. Tyner, T, Professor at California State University Fresno. Course in Introduction to Supervision of Physical Therapy Services, lecture notes, September 18, 1995.
16. A supervisor asks: "Delegation's downside." *Health Care Supervisor.* 1991;10(2):78-82.
17. Visocan BJ, Herold LS, Mulchahy MJ, Scholosser MF. Job sharing in clinical nutrition management: A plan for successful implementation. *J Am Diet Assoc.* 1993; 17(10):1141-1145.

TEST YOUR SKILLS

You are a traveling therapist. You have chosen to accept a 6-month assignment at a new rural hospital. Your job is to set up the hospital's first physical therapy department, train support personnel, and ensure that the operation will run smoothly when you leave. You have unlimited use of a hydrocollator, cold packs, ultrasound, and an electrical stimulation unit. Concerning support personnel, your budget allows you to hire two staff members. You have the choice of two individuals with no prior experience who are eager to be trained as aides. They will be paid minimum wage. You may use one, or both, or you may bring the PTA with you from your clinic in your hometown. Choosing the latter option would require a 25% increase in your labor costs. To hire the PTA, you must make accommodations elsewhere or you will have to take a cut in salary.

You arrive to find a 100-bed hospital with 95% occupancy. You also have the opportunity to take outpatients with an unlimited referral list. You must choose your own caseload for the first week. Exercising the suggestions in this chapter and relying on your knowledge of time management skills, you must decide how to manage the maximum amount of patients you can while still managing to provide quality care. You are the boss; you may set your own hours. Be sure to allow time in your schedule for documentation, equipment tasks, staff organization, and communication with other health professionals. On your list of referrals and bed occupants, you find patients with the following diagnoses:

- Low back pain (5)
- Spina bifida (2)
- Spinal cord injury (3 C-5-6, 1 T-6; 1 T-12)
- Cerebral palsy (4)
- Carpal tunnel syndrome (6)
- Adhesive capsulitis-shoulder (4)
- Post-polio syndrome (2)
- Acute Parkinson's (5)
- Cerebrovascular accident (6)
- Total knee replacement (6)
- Total hip replacement (6)
- Amputations (BK 2, AK 2)
- Cystic fibrosis (1)
- Multiple sclerosis (2)
- Emphysema (2, one with osteomyelitis)
- Compound fractures (2: 1 ankle, 1 femur)

How will you plan to handle this caseload?

	Your Schedule		Support Personnel #1		Support Personnel #2		Comments and Notes
	M-W-F	T-TH	M-W-F	T-TH	M-W-F	T-TH	
8:00 am							
8:30 am							
9:00 am							
9:30 am							
10:00 am							
10:30 am							
11:00 am							
11:30 am							
12:00 pm							
12:30 pm							
1:00 pm							
1:30 pm							
2:00 pm							
2:30 pm							
3:00 pm							
3:30 pm							
4:00 pm							
4:30 pm							

CHECK YOUR RESPONSES

First, select your staff. Consider the roles, responsibilities, and supervisory requirements of physical therapist assistants and physical therapy aides. First, does your plan meet ethical and legal requirements? As the only physical therapist in this setting, how many support personnel can you legally supervise in your state? Are you willing to accept less salary? Do you have any other choices? Are there other ways of accommodating this increase in labor costs?

How can you organize patient care needs? Are there opportunities for standardized evaluations or treatments, critical pathways, or other time- and cost-saving measures? Can patients be grouped for treatments or educational classes?

What are the tasks that can *only* be performed by a physical therapist? In what capacities can support personnel assist you? What other health professionals may need to be involved with this caseload? What questions does this raise?

You should be thinking about payer sources, level of care (acute, sub-acute, outpatient), patient access to physical therapy, authorizations for treatment, institutional policies, and program development needs.

Compare your responses with those of your colleagues and discuss the rationale for your decisions.

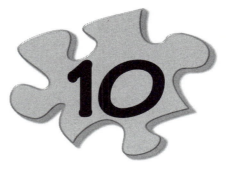

MEASURING OUTCOMES OF PHYSICAL THERAPY

Wendy Kristy, MPT

THE OUTCOMES MOVEMENT IN PHYSICAL THERAPY

To understand the outcomes movement, one needs to understand the definition of *outcome* and have a working vocabulary of terms related to this topic.

The following self-test (Table 10.1) is designed to give the reader a fundamental understanding of the terminology important in this chapter.

HISTORY OF THE OUTCOMES MOVEMENT

In reviewing the evolution of health care policy in the United States, it is easy to see that economic and political influences have shaped health care priorities. The evolution of health care has been described in three stages by AS Relman. These stages are known as the *Era of Expansion*, *Era of Cost Containment*, and *Era of Assessment and Accountability* (Figure 10.1).[2]

Era of Expansion

The Era of Expansion began at the end of World War II and continued through the 1960s. This was a time when the federal deficit was minimal and the rate of inflation was low. National priorities at this time were to annihilate disease, enhance access to health care, and end the perceived shortage of

TABLE 10.1

A SELF-TEST ON OPERATIONAL DEFINITIONS

1. What are outcomes?
   a.   A way to measure physiological improvements on a patient
   b.   Changes in health status that are attributed to care
   c.   The cost of treating a patient
   d.   The aftermath of a specific treatment protocol

2. True or False
Functional outcomes are measurable by a physical therapist, are meaningful and practical to the patient, and are economical and efficient in the eyes of payers.

3. Clinical outcomes are
   a.   An objective view of a patient's status
   b.   Test results such as range of motion, force production, manual muscle test, and the score on a pain scale
   c.   The effect of a treatment protocol on a patient
   d.   Both a and b

4. True or False
Outcomes research are studies that use cumulative data from past and ongoing treatments to determine patient outcomes.

5. True or False
Outcomes evaluation is done retrospectively, whereas outcomes management is done prospectively.

6. Give an example of an area of outcomes management related to physical therapy.
(See Page 161 for answers)

physicians. Government subsidies were provided to aid these priorities, which resulted in an increased number of specialists, better technology, increased number of hospital beds, and a growing number of insurance companies reimbursing charges.

As a result, many investor-owned medical care businesses (hospital chains) appeared because of the attractive for-profit opportunities and an open-ended system of insurance payment. The Era of Expansion culminated with the enactment of the Social Security Act (Medicare and Medicaid) in 1966, which helped to provide health care to nearly 85% of Americans.

Consider the two scenarios on Pages 162 - 163 that illustrate how physical therapy has evolved over the past 15 years.

Era of Cost Containment

The atmosphere of expansion created a sharp increase in inflation. During the early 1970s, the cost of the existing health care system became unaffordable, spurring the *Era of Cost Containment*. National emphasis shifted from

TABLE 10.1 (CONTINUED)

Check Your Answers

1. b. Outcomes are changes in a person's health status that are attributed to medical care. For example, a patient who no longer experiences shooting pains down her leg after recuperating from a laminectomy has experienced an outcome attributed to her care.

2. True. Functional outcomes are meaningful and practical to the patient. Functional outcomes are also economic and efficient in reaching a desired goal. Being able to return to competitive sports activities after anterior cruciate ligament reconstruction and rehabilitation is an example of a functional outcome.

3. d. Clinical outcomes are test results, such as force production, range of motion, manual muscle testing, or pain, that give an objective view of a patient's status. For example, "knee extensor strength at discharge is 4±5," is a clinical outcome.

4. True. Outcomes research uses cumulative data from past and ongoing treatments to determine patient outcomes. This information can then be used to determine the effectiveness and efficiency of the results. An example is tracking Functional Independence Measure (FIM) scores at admission and discharge, length of stay, and total cost. These indicators can then be used to calculate efficiency and efficacy for that patient or patients with a similar diagnosis.

5. True. In short, outcomes evaluation reviews service, whereas outcomes management produces service. Outcomes evaluation is a procedure that uses outcomes data to monitor the effectiveness and the efficiency of results achieved as well as customer satisfaction. Outcomes management uses the findings from outcomes studies to make sound health care decisions. For example, an outcomes research report indicates that patients with venous stasis ulcers experienced the same outcomes if they were treated with electrical stimulation at a frequency of three times per week and if they were treated at a frequency of five times a week. An outcomes-management strategy would involve using this information to justify treating venous ulcers with electrical stimulation three times per week instead of five times per week.

6. Five areas of outcomes management related to physical therapy
1. Prevention and management of symptom manifestation
2. Consequences of disease (impairment, disability, and/or role limitation)
3. Cost-benefit analysis
4. Health-related quality of life
5. Patient satisfaction[1]

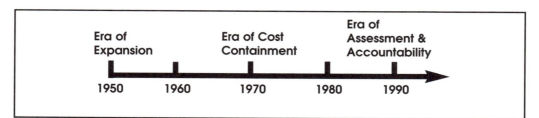

FIGURE 10.1 *Timeline of US health care trends.*

June 1983: Lisa Michaels is a new graduate from University of America's physical therapy program. She recently began her first job at a 350-bed acute medical center. She is excited to be in a stimulating, challenging health care environment as she begins her career. Her starting salary is $23,000 per year. Her caseload varies, with patients' length of stay averaging 10 to 12 days. Her patients include a young athlete who is having elective knee surgery, two elderly patients with joint replacements, a young man involved in an automobile accident with multiple fractures, a nursing home resident with a fractured hip, a new stroke patient, and one long-term patient with cancer.

She is able to work with her patients until they have achieved an independent status prior to discharge. She participates in patient rounds two to three times a week with physicians, nurses, and other caregivers, and is involved in the development and implementation of a preoperative education and postoperative transcutaneous electrical neuromuscular stimulation training program. Each week, she performs at least six new evaluations and goes home feeling as though she spent quality time with each of her patients.

June 1998: Stan Michaels, a recent graduate from University of America's physical therapy program, begins his first job at the same 350-bed medical center as Lisa. He is excited about being in a stimulating, challenging health care environment, but he does not plan to work in the hospital for more than a few years. His starting salary is $36,000 per year in addition to a $3,000 sign-on bonus. His caseload is primarily geriatric patients, with an average age of 68. His patients have multiple medical problems in addition to the condition for which they were referred for therapy. The average length of stay is now only 3 to 4 days.

Stan's caseload includes the following: a 75-year-old patient with Alzheimer's disease with a fractured hip, several patients with total knee and hip replacements, two young patients with multiple sclerosis who have been hospitalized for management of other serious medical problems, a 68-year-old patient post-coronary artery bypass who just had his second above-knee amputation, and a 45-year-old patient with quadriplegia with osteomyelitis, which resulted from an untreated pressure area. Patients now are sometimes discharged before he has a chance to instruct their families in how to assist them. Rarely does he have an opportunity to discuss a case in depth with the attending physician. Even when there is an indication that a longer length of stay is needed, he and the hospital staff are under pressure to discharge the patient to a lower level of care.

The department in which he works has experienced a high turnover rate, and there are currently several positions open. He performs 12 to 15 new evaluations per week and finds that he does not have enough time to see all of his patients himself. There is always a waiting list of referrals waiting to be seen.

continued on Page 163

Part-time, per-diem, and registry staff see all of his patients on his days off, but Stan is concerned about the discontinuity of care this creates. He leaves work feeling exhausted and discouraged that he can do so little for his patients, despite the excellent training he received in school.[3]

expansion to reorganization of the health care system with an emphasis on efficiency. This was accomplished by promoting health maintenance organizations (HMOs) and preferred provider organizations (PPOs) and by negotiating fees and discounted rates.[4]

In 1983, Medicare implemented a system of payment for acute hospitalization by diagnosis-related group (DRG), which changed reimbursement from retrospective fee-for-service payment to a prospective lump-sum payment. Essentially, the DRG system changed the reimbursement for Medicare patients in acute hospitals from payment of a bill for services rendered to a prospective payment per admission, at a rate determined by the patient's diagnosis. Changes in reimbursement demanded new strategies from both hospital-based and outpatient providers. Because of an increased financial risk, providers began negotiating contracts with payers, competing with each other for health care dollars.[4]

Era of Assessment and Accountability

Three factors led to the *Era of Assessment and Accountability*:
1. The need for cost containment.
2. A renewed sense of competition.
3. The work of researchers who performed successful outcomes studies.

According to Arnold Epstein, researchers who performed successful outcome studies were the most significant influence leading to the Era of Assessment and Accountability.[5] During the early 1980s, one of these researchers (John Wennberg) documented substantial geographic differences in the use of various medical procedures.[6,7] These differences persisted even after controlling for severity of illness. This was disturbing information, and questions followed concerning whether these variations reflected unnecessary costs in high-use areas or less-than-optimal care in low-use areas.

Needless to say, outcomes research was the first step to answer these questions. As a result of Wennberg's research, the US Congress became attentive to outcomes data, and Wennberg became a powerful advocate for using scientific evidence to make health care decisions.[6]

Outcomes data is the key to making sound clinical decisions, and enhances quality patient care and cost efficiency.[8]

The Era of Assessment and Accountability essentially began in 1988, when the Health Care Financing Administration sponsored an invitational conference. At this conference, representatives from government, private insurers, major corporations, community agencies, and the medical profession met to discuss the need for assessment and accountability.[2]

It was unanimously agreed that outcomes data were necessary to understand the variations in performance among providers to create a basis for funding future health care. It was also agreed that more needs to be known about the relative costs, safety, and effectiveness of all the things physicians do or employ in the diagnosis, treatment, and prevention of disease.[2]

The outcomes movement has changed our focus from a "process" to an actual "product." Today, outcomes data are currently being used in physical therapy (and general medicine) to develop consensus statements, practice guidelines, and practice protocols. Furthermore, these data are being offered as standards for third-party reimbursement and malpractice protection. Therefore, understanding the roots of the outcomes movement may shed light on the current practice trends of the day.[5,9] "Health policy decisions will increasingly be based on outcome studies of health-related quality of life."[10]

ORGANIZATIONS ACTIVE IN THE OUTCOMES MOVEMENT

Accreditation Organizations

These organizations contribute to the quality of care provided in hospitals and rehabilitation facilities. By using outcomes data, these organizations provide standards for facility accreditation, which in turn enhance quality of care provided.

Joint Commission on Accreditation of Health Care Organizations

The organization for hospital accreditation is known as the Joint Commission on Accreditation of Health Care Organizations (JCAHO). JCAHO was formed in 1951 when the American College of Physicians, the American Hospital Association, and the American Medical Association joined with the American College of Surgeons to set minimum hospital standards. Prior to this (1917-1951), only the American College of Surgeons had been setting hospital standards. Today, JCAHO uses information from top US health care experts to provide guidelines for hospital and institutional accreditation. These guidelines include the required number and mix of staff members in each unit, area, and department to provide for patient needs.[11]

Commission on Accreditation of Rehabilitation Facilities

The accrediting organization for rehabilitation facilities is known as the Commission on Accreditation of Rehabilitation Facilities (CARF). CARF has been in existence for the past 20 years.[12] Its standards are used for accreditation of rehabilitation facilities and are based on severity-adjusted outcomes (outcomes of groups who vary by severity of disability). To accomplish its mission, CARF provides guidelines for facility utilization and qualified personnel.

Agency for Health Care Policy and Research

The Agency for Health Care Policy and Research was created in 1989 specifically to fund research that emphasized the effectiveness and appropriateness of health care services and procedures. This was done by assessing outcomes, which provided information regarding which clinical interventions are most beneficial.

These outcome assessment activities, known as the Medical Treatment Effectiveness Program, use databases similar to those used by the Medicare program. Today, patient outcomes research teams (PORTs) have also been created to explore practice patterns and costs of care, and to store up information on patient outcomes. Later in this chapter, some recent outcomes studies done by PORT researchers are summarized.[13]

DISABLEMENT MODELS

Disablement refers to the various conditions of function that affect basic human performance and social roles. The disablement models in this section are presented to help the reader understand some concepts that can help guide specifications for program outcomes.

Two Models of Disablement

World Health Organization

The World Health Organization (WHO) provides a disablement scheme called the International Classification of Impairments, Disabilities and Handicaps (ICIDH). This scheme is used for disability policy planning, statistics, and clinical management worldwide, although it is not well-known in the United States. The WHO defines impairment, disability, and handicap as follows:

- Impairment is a loss or abnormality at the organ level (ie, amputation of a limb or loss of hip extension).
- Disability is the inability to function as expected for a human being at the person's level (ie, difficulty walking or climbing stairs).
- Handicap is the disadvantage resulting from the interaction of the impairment or disability with the person's environment (ie, not being able to get into one's third-floor office).[8,14]

Nagi scheme

In comparison, the Nagi scheme offers the following slightly different definitions:

- Impairment is an anatomical, physiological, mental, or emotional abnormality or loss.
- Functional limitation is a limitation in performance at the level of the whole person.
- Disability is the limitation in performance of socially defined roles and tasks within a socio-cultural and physical environment.[14]

In an effort to define a common vocabulary for all health care entities to use when referring to disablement, Nagi and WHO have developed models of disablement (Table 10.2). Outcomes researchers can use these models as a way to help define and understand program outcomes.

When considering the Nagi and ICIDH models of disablement, it appears they are very similar in their definitions of active pathology, disease, and impairment. However, there are some differences in their views of the consequences of disease and pathology. For example, Nagi considers disability to be a "limitation in the performance of socially defined roles..." whereas the WHO/ICIDH model considers this definition to be a handicap. Despite the differences in these models, we can use them to illustrate the role of physical therapy in the disablement scheme.

As physical therapists, we have traditionally focused on reducing our patient's "impairment" and have addressed the patient's function at an "organ system level" (ie, increasing range of motion). However, many times, the goals for our patients in rehabilitation are long-term maintenance and gradual integration into family and community roles. Therefore, instead of focusing our treatment on impairments, we should focus on reducing the patient's "disability" or "handicap" (ie, getting a patient back to his or her full work responsibilities). Consider the scenario on Page 167.

TABLE 10.2

MODELS OF DISABLEMENT

Nagi Scheme

Active pathology	Impairment	Functional limitation	Disability
Interruption or interference with normal processes and efforts of the organism to regain a normal state	Anatomical, physiological, mental, or emotional abnormalities or loss	Limitation in performance at the level of the whole organism or person	Limitation in performance, of socially defined roles and tasks within a socio-cultural and physical environment

International Classification of Impairment, Disabilities, and Handicaps (ICIDH)

Disease	Impairment	Disability	Handicap
The intrinsic pathology of disorder—anatomical	Loss or abnormality of psychological, structure, or function at the organ level	Restriction or ability to perform an activity in the normal manner	Disadvantage, impairment or disability that limits or prevents fulfillment of a normal role (depends on age, sex, socio-economic factors) for the person

Reprinted from Jette AM. Physical disablement concepts for physical therapy research and practice. Phys Ther. 1994;74(5):380-386, with permission from the APTA.

Samuel Blevens is a 38-year-old carpenter who has experienced severe back pain since being in a car accident 1 week ago. Upon evaluation at Getwell Physical Therapy, you find that he has severe pain with sitting and standing for long periods of time, as well as with lifting and twisting. His pain sometimes radiates down the front of his thighs to his knees. He has been unable to work or drive since the accident, and he is unable to care for his live-in mother. Your physical examination revealed that he has a thoracolumbar spine scoliosis with muscle spasms and tenderness in the surrounding areas. He is also limited to only 25% of flexion, extension, rotation, and side bending in all directions.

Using the ICIDH definitions, you could identify Mr. Blevens' pain, decreased lumbosacral spine range of motion (into spinal flexion, extension, rotation, and side bending), and muscle spasm as impairments. His disabilities include not being able to drive, sit, or stand at home or at work for long periods of time. His handicap, or social disadvantage, would include not being able to work or care for his mother.

To reduce a patient's handicap, goals for our patients should reflect their expected outcomes. In the case of Mr. Blevens, long-term goals should include returning to a productive work role and possibly modifying his environment (ie, work, home) and the ways he functions within those environments. Achieving these goals may be a considerable challenge and requires collaboration with community resources and his workplace. Yet, those programs that produce positive outcomes (ie, those outcomes that extend beyond impairment) will have an edge in competing for managed care contracts.[12]

Disablement models help us to see the advantage of examining the potential benefits of physical therapy in achieving outcomes related to a patient's disability, as well as outcomes related to his or her impairments. Some researchers suggest that there is a linear relationship between impairments, disabilities, and handicaps, inferring that changes in an impairment result in predictable changes in disabilities and handicaps. However, according to Jette, this linear relationship does not always exist for at least two reasons.[8]

First, consider the force production of a muscle and the reduction of a disability. The increase in a muscle's force production does not always reduce disability. For example, a patient who demonstrates a 5/5 manual muscle test in his or her lower extremities may not necessarily be able to walk. Therefore, there is more to function than just force production, such as sensation, coordination, and balance. Analyzing the relationship of function and muscle force production shows a threshold point in which further force production does not increase function (Figure 10.2).

Secondly, many factors affect the relationship between impairment and function. The degree to which an increase in force production improves disability also depends on factors such as the individual's psychological response to the injury, the attitudes of significant others in the patient's social networks, and the patient's physical environment.[8]

This complex relationship between impairment and disability has not been studied extensively in traditional clinical research. We must understand that the role of physical therapy in rehabilitation is to reduce a patient's disability and handicap and not only to address his or her impairments. We need clinical outcomes research that addresses both impairment and disabilities, and the relationship existing between them across various target groups.[8]

OUTCOMES TODAY

As providers, we are continually being asked to do more for less, a trend that many fear may threaten the quality of health care and thereby our nation's health status. Therefore, in order to measure up to what we are

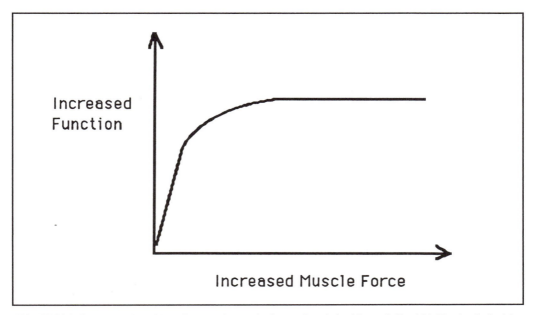

FIGURE 10.2 *Relationship of function and muscle force. Reprinted from Jette AM. Physical disablement concepts for physical therapy research and practice. Phys Ther. 1994; 74(5):380-386, with permission from the APTA.*

expected to do, we need to analyze what has worked best in the past. A way to do this is through outcomes research—a system for analyzing different indicators and patterns that may lead us toward more effective and cost-efficient treatments.

Common indicators can be tracked for patients with similar diagnoses and then analyzed to determine the outcome (ie, cost, quality, patient satisfaction) (Table 10.3). If done prospectively (in a data collection system designed with this in mind), a growing database of valuable information can be created. This information can then be used to benefit not only the provider, but patients and payers as well.

However, not all agree that outcomes research is valid information. Consider the following scenario:

George Sandwall, a staff physical therapist at Blanchfield Rehabilitation, decides to do an outcomes study on patient satisfaction using a Likert scale. The scale is ordinal, with 1 being "strongly disagree" and 5 being "strongly agree." With some patients (50%) extremely satisfied and others who are extremely dissatisfied (15%), he decides to average the scores. The result is an average of 4.3.

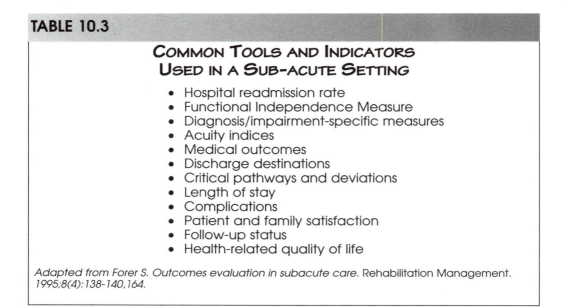

TABLE 10.3

COMMON TOOLS AND INDICATORS
USED IN A SUB-ACUTE SETTING

- Hospital readmission rate
- Functional Independence Measure
- Diagnosis/impairment-specific measures
- Acuity indices
- Medical outcomes
- Discharge destinations
- Critical pathways and deviations
- Length of stay
- Complications
- Patient and family satisfaction
- Follow-up status
- Health-related quality of life

Adapted from Forer S. Outcomes evaluation in subacute care. Rehabilitation Management. *1995;8(4):138-140,164.*

Insurers might be very impressed with this seemingly great outcome. Unfortunately, it is not an accurate interpretation of the data and, therefore, may not be comparable to other patient groups or other institutions using the same scale. Averaging ordinal data, as in the scores from a Likert scale, is inappropriate. A more appropriate way to analyze these data would be to calculate the percentage of the subjects who marked each of the criteria. For example, 85% of patients said they strongly agreed that they were greeted as soon as they came in the door. Only 2% reported that they disagreed or strongly disagreed that they were greeted as they came in the door.

Another problem with outcomes data concerns external validity. Because we are unable to control the many variables that contribute to the outcome, such as a patient's diagnosis, prior medical history, and the physician's decision-making process, the outcomes of one patient may not be comparable to another patient with a similar diagnosis.

Such threats to external validity limit the generalizability of the findings of a particular study to a population. Therefore, acceptable methods to control and report database research must be employed. Choosing an appropriate sampling method and controlling for variables such as age, prior level of function, social support, co-morbidity, and planning prospective studies are important strategies for facilities attempting to perform outcomes studies.

Bridgette Ames is a 55-year-old school librarian who had been experiencing increased arthritic pain in her left hip. She had progressed to the point where she had extreme difficulty with sitting, walking, and sleeping, and was faced with having to quit her part-time position with the school district. She had been seeing an orthopedic specialist off and on for the past 5 years for this problem. At her last visit, her doctor said he felt she would benefit from a total hip arthroplasty. Hopeful of relieving her pain, Ms. Ames agreed to undergo the surgery.

After the surgery, she spent 5 days in the hospital and then was discharged home to her family. While in the hospital, she received daily physical therapy treatments. After 2 weeks of recuperation at home, she came into the outpatient physical therapy clinic for therapeutic exercise once per week for 4 weeks. Eight weeks postoperatively, Ms. Ames rented a wheelchair to simplify her mobility on the job and returned to work. Now, 1 year later, she feels as though the surgery made "all the difference in the world." She had returned to work full-time and was independent in all her activities of daily living. Ms. Ames' total cost of care was $25,000.

Compare the outcome of Ms. Ames with the following case:

Carlos Hernandez is a 58-year-old uninsured, migrant farm worker. He has a history of hypertension and diabetes and has developed a mild peripheral neuropathy in his legs and hands. One year ago, he slipped and fell in a wet parking lot and sustained a hip fracture. He was taken to the local county hospital via ambulance where he had a hemiarthroplasty performed. Two days after his surgery, he had a stroke, which necessitated treatment in the intensive care unit for 1 week, followed by 2 more weeks in the acute hospital. He then stayed 2 months in a rehabilitation hospital before going home, where he received 2 more months of home health physical therapy. Mr. Hernandez is no longer able to work, and he requires assistance with personal hygiene, dressing, transfers, ambulation, and eating. Total cost of care for Mr. Hernandez thus far is $200,000.

As you can see from these two scenarios, a similar procedure can have vastly different outcomes. There are many factors that dictate the outcome of each individual patient. Mr. Hernandez' pre-morbid condition put him at risk for a less desirable outcome (ie, stroke, loss of livelihood and independence, higher cost care, and lowered quality of life). Ms. Ames' pre-morbid condition had fewer risks, and she realized a very positive outcome (ie, full independence). With careful consideration, an outcomes database can be programmed to account for these differences and, therefore, allow us to more accurately compare results in similar cases.

The different outcomes for Mr. Hernandez and Ms. Ames are important and must be addressed when evaluating outcomes data. We should also be concerned that many current decisions we make as health professionals and payers are based on evidence that has not been scientifically tested. To date, many protocols and practice decisions we use are based on the general consensus of professionals with experience in the topic area. However, data from outcomes research can only enhance our decision-making abilities and, thus, improve the quality of care that we provide.

OUTCOMES TOOLS

Understanding the Basics

A Guide to Physical Therapist Practice gives a description of five patient outcomes that can be used to measure the influence of physical therapy intervention.[1] These outcomes are:
- Prevention and management of symptom manifestation
- Consequences of disease (impairment, disability, and/or role limitation)
- Cost-benefit analysis
- Health-related quality of life
- Patient satisfaction

By using an outcomes database, patient information can easily be extracted to compute the desired information. Depending on the parameters or indicators used in the database, information concerning the outcomes above can be analyzed. This information is extremely valuable to our decision-making abilities as health professionals and allows us to evaluate the efficiency and efficacy of the care we provide.

Outcomes evaluation provides many benefits to the user, including the following:
- Identification of problem areas requiring more detailed investigation
- Better alignment of goals and objectives with client needs
- Availability of outcomes data for research purposes
- Information on cost effectiveness

"Despite these inherent benefits, most sub-acute (and outpatient) providers have not engaged in outcomes evaluation. This may be due in part to the lack of well-defined and tested outcomes measures that are appropriate for sub-acute care."[15]

To understand outcomes data, the clinician must be comfortable with research design and data analysis methods. These areas have not been a priority for many clinicians and students. Yet, now that the health care environment is demanding outcomes data, those clinicians who are comfortable with research design and data analysis methods will have an edge on the outcomes market.

Currently, outcomes have been tracked primarily for inpatient care but not as widely for outpatient care. According to JP Reynolds, no matter the type or size of a physical therapy practice, outcomes need to be tracked.[9] For data to be useful to both the practitioner and the external community (such as the insurance companies who pay you), the data need to be interpreted.

"Boring," you may say. Some fundamental elements of statistics and research design to understand include the following:

- Measures of central tendency (mean, median, mode)
- Standard deviation
- Data types (nominal, ordinal, interval, and ratio)
- Statistical tests appropriate for specific data types
- Concepts of measurement: validity and reliability
- Concepts of value: efficiency and efficacy
- Differences between clinical and experimental research

This information can easily be obtained at most universities and colleges. Also, collaborating with someone knowledgeable in these areas can help clinicians work with outcomes data.[9]

The hospital where you work uses a database system that allows for indicators to be tracked and analyzed statistically. The data from the last two quarters indicate that an increasing number of diabetic wound patients were denied reimbursement for treatment in the past 6 months. The board of directors has asked you, manager of the rehabilitation services department, to give a report on the cost efficiency of your two wound care protocols for pressure ulcers (total contact casting and whirlpool/debridement).

COLLECTING OUTCOMES DATA

To accomplish this task, you must first determine what information you need to calculate cost efficiency of wound care. Questions to consider include, "What indicators do I track?" and "How do I control for co-morbidity?"

You decide to use the following categories as indicators for your outcomes report:
- Number of visits
- Cost of supplies
- Cost of services
- Type of dressing
- Initial wound size
- Length of treatment
- Pre-existing health conditions
- Age

With the data collected from these categories, a series of numbers are generated, and now you are faced with interpreting them. With your database, you extract and analyze the data, which is summarized in Table 10.4.

Table 10.4 illustrates there is a quicker healing rate in the total contact casting (TCC) method. On average, TCC produced wound closure within 24 weeks; whereas, the whirlpool/debridement (W/D) method produced wound closure in 32 weeks.

The data also showed that supplies were three times more expensive for TCC than W/D (ie, $300 per TCC visit versus $100 per W/D treatment); however, TCC patients are seen only twice per month as opposed to twice per week for W/D patients.

Key calculations:
- Cost per visit = cost of supplies/visit + cost of services/visit
- Average total cost = number of visits x cost per visit

Average total cost for the TCC method was $4200. Average total costs for the W/D method was $9600.

Your outcomes report indicates that the TCC method of treatment cost $5400 less than the W/D method of treatment, making it the more cost-effective treatment.

Much of your success here will depend on what types of instruments you use, how you use them, and whether you decide to become part of a national database.[9] There are companies that will provide you with the software to collect your data; then, for a fee, the company will run the data analysis for you.

TABLE 10.4

OUTCOMES REPORT

	Total contact casting	Whirlpool/ debridement
Cost of supplies per visit	$350	$100
Average frequency of visits per week	0.5	2.0
Physical therapy charge per visit	$50	$50
Average healing time (weeks)	24	32
Total cost per visit	$350	$150
Average total cost to heal wound	$4200	$9600

This is helpful if you happen to want the specific information analyzed by your service. However, you may need to have more flexibility with your data analysis so that you can identify and track other trends in your outcomes.

Outcomes Databases

Starting an outcomes database is no easy task, and it would be wise to investigate existing programs before implementing a new system. Because assessing outcomes is a research problem, it is important to have the data evaluated by someone who has expertise in the area of research methods as well as rehabilitation.[16] Some prerequisites to generating outcomes data include having a computer, knowing what questions you want to ask, and having a grasp of research design and statistics. Several resources are available that offer information and guidance on choosing an appropriate instrument. Some of these resources offer a comparative description of a wide variety of standardized tests.

APTA's Research, Analysis, and Development Division has gathered information on nonprofit computerized databases. Two of them are listed here: the National Pain Data Bank and the Uniform Data System for Medical Rehabilitation.[9]

The National Pain Data Bank

The National Pain Data Bank was developed by the American Academy of Pain Management and contains information on roughly 3600 patients treated for pain. Information is taken at intake, discharge, and follow-up regarding demographics, patient history, pain profile, return to work, functional status, quality of life, patient satisfaction, and cost of care. Quarterly data comparison reports are provided to those who belong to the data bank.

Uniform Data Set for Medical Rehabilitation (UDSMR)

The Uniform Data Set for Medical Rehabilitation, created in 1983, is one of the first rehabilitation outcomes databases. More than 700 rehabilitation facilities are a part of the Uniform Data Set, which contains more that one million patient records. Facilities that join this database are tested and trained to use the outcomes tools (Functional Independence Measure [FIM] and Functional Independence Measure of Children [WeeFIM]). The software package, *FIMware*, is also included. This program graphically represents change in patients' functional status over time and allows 45 data fields for optional use by the facility. For more information, write to UDSMR Data Management Service; 232 Parker Hall; 3435 Main Street; Buffalo, NY 14214; fax: (716) 829-2080; phone (716) 829-2076.

The FIM is one of many objective measures used to score patients' function at various times during their rehabilitation (ie, prior, admission, goal, weekly/monthly, discharge, and follow-up). Basic scoring is as follows, but may be modified to accommodate the needs of the setting.

No Help Needed

(7 points) Complete independence (timely, safely)

(6 points) Modified independence (device needed or extra time needed)

Helper Needed

(5 points) Supervision (stand by assistance)

(4 points) Minimal assistance (75% work by patient)

(3 points) Moderate assistance (50% work by patient)

(2 points) Maximal assistance (25% work by patient)

(1 point) Total assistance (0% work by patient)

These FIM levels can be used to score a patient's functional status in areas such as transfers (bed, chair, wheelchair, toilet, tub, shower), locomotion (walking, wheelchair mobility, stairs), and bed mobility (rolling, scooting, supine to sit transfer). Other areas may also include self-care, bowel/bladder management, and communication.

Vencare is one of many companies that provide contracted rehabilitation services to skilled nursing facilities nationwide. Vencare uses a tracking system that captures more than 200,000 interactions between clinicians and patients each month. At year-end 1997, this system contained data on more than 85,000 patients. Their clinical documentation system (TheraSys) forces the clinical team to focus care on the return of the functional life skills of the patient[18] by using the FIM. FIM scores are determined at the initial evaluation (weekly and at discharge) and are used for statistical analysis to determine the most appropriate, cost-effective care plan as well as the amount of staffing required to achieve the desired outcome. With this computerized clinical decision support, the individual clinical manager is able to compare individual patients with thousands of other patients with similar diagnoses and levels of disablement. In addition, graphic presentations of the outcomes are used to communicate with physicians, hospital discharge planners, and other caregivers in the community to demonstrate the effectiveness of treatment in returning patients to a functional level.[18]

Commercial Providers of Outcomes Services

Focus on Therapeutic Outcomes

The following services are offered by Focus on Therapeutic Outcomes, Inc (FOTO, Inc), an example of a commercial provider of therapeutic outcomes services:

FOTO, Inc, provides outcomes data collection and report services across the rehabilitation continuum. We offer standardized measurement instruments, which are patient focused, easy to use, statistically valid, clinically appropriate, cost effective and efficient. Our reports are risk adjusted, which offers FOTO providers a "fair and level" playing field for national benchmarking and data comparison. We are a service company and we fully understand that role. We pride ourselves in quality products and timely response to our clients' needs and requests.

The procedure is as simple and noninvasive as possible. We understand the documentation overload in the clinic, and we strive hard to minimize the impact of collecting this valuable information. The intake involves obtaining functional and demographic information from the patient mostly and from the staff minimally. The same information is taken from the patient at discharge. The information required from the staff at discharge is the demographic and functional data normally collected in rehabilitation. In addition to reports, which are distributed quarterly, our comparative reports include comparative functional outcome indexes, or the average functional change per episode, per dollar spent, and per visit.[19]

OUTCOMES STUDIES

As mentioned earlier, the Agency for Health Care Policy and Research funds outcomes research. PORTs have been created to explore practice patterns, costs of care, and to store information on patient outcomes. Recently, the Total Knee Replacement (TKR) PORT studied TKR outcomes. Its purpose was to concentrate on assessing and improving the outcomes of the TKR procedure. Three of their studies are summarized here as examples of outcomes research.[20]

1.   Culler SD, Holmes AM, Gutierres B. Expected hospital costs of knee replacement for rural residents by locations of services. *Medical Care*. 1995;33(12):1188-1209. This study analyzed data from 1985 to 1989 from HCFA's *Medicare Provider Analysis and Review*.

   They found that the predicted cost of total knee replacements is less in rural hospitals than in urban hospitals, particularly those hospitals that do more than nine of these procedures per year. Cost savings ranged from $1560 to $6306 (depending on severity of illness and number of knee replacements). It was found that by increasing a hospital's volume even by one knee replacement per year, the predicted cost per case fell. This incremental savings decreased as volume increased, although cost savings remained higher in rural hospitals compared to urban hospitals. These data support the regionalization of services, especially in rural areas.

2.   Wright J, Heck D, Hawker G, et al. Rates of tibial osteotomies in Canada and the United States. *Clinical Orthopaedics*. 1995;226-275.

   This study compares osteotomy and TKR rates in both Ontario, Canada, and the United States from 1985 to 1990 using HCFA, Ontario Health Insurance Plan, and National Hospital Discharge Survey databases. It found that the rates of osteotomies declined 11% to 14% per year in patients 65 years and older and by 3% to 4% per year in patients younger than 65. Men received twice as many osteotomies as women in both countries. Osteotomies in the United States were two to three times lower than in Ontario. The reason for the decline of osteotomies was attributed to the growing rate of TKR procedures and surgeons' growing confidence in TKR outcomes. However, the lack of difference in rates of osteotomies in younger individuals can be attributed to the advantages of this procedure for the younger age group. Osteotomy lessens pain in roughly 80% of patients, and in most cases, allows patients to return to vigorous sports activities. However, the pain relief is generally incomplete and returns to previous levels in 50% of patients. Therefore, tibial osteotomies may be the viable choice for younger, more active individuals wanting to return to vigorous activities, but not for the older patient. For younger patients, prosthetic longevity becomes an issue because the likelihood of requiring a new prosthesis is high. TKRs are the preferred choice for older patients because vigorous activity and longevity of prostheses are generally of less concern.

3.   Hawker G, Melfi C, Paul J, et al. Comparison of a generic (SF-36) and a disease specific (WOMAC) instrument in the measure of outcomes after knee replacement surgery. *J Rheumatol*. 1995;22(6):1193-1196.

In this study, the TKR PORT investigators compared the generic health-related quality of life (HRQL) measure (SF-36) with the Western Ontario and McMaster Universities Osteoarthritis Index (WOMAC), a disease-specific HRQL measure. It assessed the health status of nearly 1200 Medicare patients who had undergone knee replacement surgery 2 to 7 years previously. The data were accumulated through a mail survey to randomized samples of Medicare beneficiaries. The researchers concluded that generic measures are necessary to compare outcomes across different populations and different diseases, whereas disease-specific measures assess the specific disabilities of patients in defined diagnostic groups.

STRATEGIES TO PREPARE FOR CHANGE

Some strategies to help you operate better in the world of outcomes include the following:

Educate Yourself

Read and study *A Guide to Physical Therapist Practice,*[1] This document is an invaluable source of information that all physical therapy students should read and study. It offers comprehensive insight into the world of patient management, patient examination, and intervention.

Additionally, the reader can find the *Guidelines for Physical Therapy Documentation, Standards of Practice for Physical Therapy,* and the *Guide for Professional Conduct of the American Physical Therapy Association* included in Appendices 2, 3, and 4. These documents will give you a clearer understanding of your roles as a physical therapist.[21]

Understand Documentation

Being familiar with payer needs and utilization review will help you to avoid the usual pitfalls in documentation. Also, by being more focused on functional outcomes and less focused on impairment outcomes, we can help show reviewers that our treatments lead to functional outcomes. More information on this topic will be covered in Chapter 12.[22]

Understand Research Design and Rudimentary Statistics

As illustrated earlier, understanding research design is imperative to prosper in the outcomes movement. Increase your level of comfort with basic differences between clinical and experimental research, efficiency and efficacy, and validity and reliability. Also, gain a clear understanding of data analysis

TABLE 10.5

WORDS FOR THE WISE

1. **Collaborate**
   For those who lack the expertise to develop appropriate outcomes questions or analyze data, collaboration with researchers is imperative. Consulting with a physical therapy education program or a local statistician is a good place to start.
2. **Educate the administration**
   If you understand the basics of research, you can help your supervisor understand the steps needed for outcomes data collection and analysis.
3. **Use your resources**
   Consult the literature through public and hospital libraries. Another good resource is Medline, which is accessible at many hospital libraries. Also, you can access many university catalogues on the Internet.[9]

methods (measures of central tendency, means and standard deviation, frequency distributions, and other statistical tests).

Without this knowledge, we are limited in our decision-making abilities and, therefore, we are at a disadvantage when it comes to competing for contracts with third-party payers.[9,21] The better educated we are in these areas, the better are our abilities to operate in a rapidly changing health care environment. Table 10.5 lists some steps physical therapists can take to incorporate outcomes management into their daily practice.

Utilizing Technology

Implementing a database system is an easy way to track outcomes. Such a system can greatly increase the speed of documentation, outcomes analysis, as well as make an organization more competitive in the managed care environment.

However, installing such a system is no easy task. It has been predicted that for many health care providers, expenditures on information technology will probably need to increase 300% to 400% within 5 years to create high-quality systems.[23]

If you find yourself part of an organization that is considering implementing a database (ie, computerized documentation), you should consider the readiness of your staff to adapt to change. Only with a full commitment at the executive level and a shared vision with the employees will such an endeavor succeed. It is wise to consult with others about which database is best for your practice. The tools used for measuring functional outcomes need to be proven reliable and valid. A list of resources for information on outcomes instruments is mentioned previously in this chapter. For further information on how to implement an outcomes database, contact APTA's Department of Practice at (800) 999-APTA or visit their website. (http://www.apta.org).

Critical Indicators

Give considerable thought as to which indicators you will use when tracking data. Outcomes data are used for developing consensus statements, practice guidelines, and treatment protocols, as well as being offered as standards for third-party reimbursement and malpractice protection. Because there are so many groups that are interested in outcomes, you will need to customize your data analysis to meet your needs.

Total Quality Management

Total quality management (TQM) is a movement that is gaining momentum as patient satisfaction and quality services are balancing out the focus on cutting costs. Outcomes data can help to improve the quality of services and determine cost-efficiency—two important entities of TQM (see Chapter 13). Quality of service can be improved by using outcomes data to set practice standards, design critical pathways, and enhance decision making. Cost efficiency can be identified by tracking indicators such as length of stay, patient satisfaction, and cost of care (see Table 10.4).

RESOURCES FOR MORE INFORMATION ABOUT OUTCOMES INSTRUMENTS

1. Basmajian J, ed. *Physical Rehabilitation Outcomes Measures.* Toronto: Canadian Physiotherapy Association, Health and Welfare Canada, and Canada Communications Group; 1994.
2. Lewis C, McNerney T. *The Functional Tool Box.* Washington DC: Learn Publications; 1994.
3. McDowell I, Newell C. *Measuring Health, 2nd Ed.* New York: Oxford University Press; 1996.
4. Rossetti L. *Infant-Toddler Assessment.* New York: Oxford University Press; 1996.
5. Stewart D, Abeln SH. *Documenting Functional Outcomes in Physical Therapy.* St. Louis, Mo: Mosby-Year Book Inc; 1993.
6. Physical Disability. Special Issue. *Phys Ther.* 1994; 74:375-503.

Reprinted from Reynolds JP. Outcomes: all the data in the world. PT-Magazine of Physical Therapy. 1996; 4(7):48-53, with permission from the American Physical Therapy Association.

REFERENCES

1. American Physical Therapy Association. *A Guide to Physical Therapist Practice.* Alexandria, Va: American Physical Therapy Association; 1997.
2. Relman AS. Assessment and accountability: the third revolution in medical care. *N Engl J Med.* 1988;319(18):1220-1222.
3. Curtis KA, Martin T. Recruitment and retention in acute care. *Rehab Management.* 1991;4(5):69-76.
4. Stewart DL, Abeln SH. *Documenting Functional Outcomes in Physical Therapy.* St. Louis, MO: Mosby-Year Book, Inc.; 1993.
5. Reynolds JP. What is the outcomes movement? what it means to PTs. *PT-Magazine of Physical Therapy.* 1995;3(7):49-52, 67-68.
6. Epstein AM. Sounding board: the outcomes movement—will it get us where we want to go? *N Engl J Med.* 1990;323(4):266-270.
7. Wennberg J, Gittelsohn A. Small-area variations in health care delivery. *Science.* 1973;182:1102-1108.
8. Jette AM. Outcomes research; shifting the dominant research paradigm in physical therapy. *Phys Ther.* 1995;75:965-970.
9. Reynolds JP. Outcomes: all the data in the world. *PT-Magazine of Physical Therapy.* 1996;4(7):48-50, 52-53.
10. Jenkins CD. Assessment of outcomes of health intervention. *Social Science and Medicine.* 1992;35(3-4):367.
11. Roberts JS, Coale JG, Redman RR. A history of the Joint Commission of Accreditation of Hospitals. *JAMA.* 1987; 258(7): 936-940.
12. Wilkerson D. Developing outcomes management tools. *Rehab Management.* 1995;8(1):114-117, 129.
13. Benjamin K. Outcomes research and the allied health professional. *J Allied Health.* 1995;24(1):3-12.
14. Jette AM. Physical disablement concepts for physical therapy research and practice. *Phys Ther.* 1994;74(5):380-386.
15. Forer S. Outcomes evaluation in subacute care. *Rehab Management.* 1995;8(4):138-140.
16. Moore RW, Salcido R. Rehabilitation outcomes in subacute care. *Rehab Management.* 1996;9(1):97-111.
17. Reynolds JP. Outcomes: all the data in the world. *PT-Magazine of Physical Therapy.* 1996; 4(7):48-53.
18. Vencare Ancillary Services. *Positioning the future of postacute services: rehab overview year-end 1997.* Louisville, Ky: VenCare Health Services; 1998.
19. *Focus on Therapeutic Outcomes, What We Do.* Knoxville, TN: FOTO Inc, 1998. http://www.fotoinc.com/press.htm, 6/30/98.
20. AHCPR. Total knee replacement PORT publishes recent findings. *AHCPR.* 1996;194(96-0061):8-9.
21. Lisa Culver, Associate Director of APTA's Department of Practice. Phone interview on September 27, 1996.
22. Cohn R. Managed care in intermediate care settings part 1: Implications and strategies. *PT-Magazine od Physical Therapy.* 1996;4(7):28-31.
23. Meleski BW. Evolving information culture. *PT-Magazine of Physical Therapy.* 1996; 4(6):42-44.

TEST YOUR SKILLS

1. Discuss the perspective of each of the following parties on this patient's outcomes:
    a. Patient
    b. Physical therapist
    c. Employer
    d. Payer

Lance is a 33-year-old mail carrier who strained his back 6 months ago at work while lifting a 60-pound box. Workers' compensation insurance covers his rehabilitation on a fee-for-service basis. The US Postal Service pays $350 per month per employee for Workers' compensation insurance, in addition to Lance's $30,000 per year salary, and an additional $12,000 per year for Lance's part-time replacement. After 2 weeks of intensive physical therapy, Lance returned to work on light duty, not being able to lift more than 15 pounds. After 2 months of light duty and twice per week physical therapy visits (averaging $100 per visit), he progressed to his regular work duties, only to re-injure his back 2 weeks later. After taking 3 days off, he returned to work on light duty again. Now, 3 months later, he still has not progressed to lifting more that 15 pounds despite his physical therapy visits twice per week.

a. Patient

b. Physical therapist

c. Employer

d. Payer

2.   Consider the following two scenarios.

Case 1

Salazar is a 38-year-old man who strained his back while lifting a heavy box at work. His doctor referred him to facility A for physical therapy, where he was seen 10 times at $40 per visit. At his first visit, he scored 45/100 on the lumbar spine Functional Rating Scale (FRS). At discharge, he scored 98/100. Within 8 weeks, Salazar returned to work full-time without restrictions.

Case 2

Harrison is a 41-year-old man who strained his back in a car accident. His doctor referred him to facility B, where he was seen seven times at $60 per visit. At his first visit, he scored 45/100 on the lumbar spine FRS. At discharge, he scored 90/100. Within 6 weeks, Harrison was able to return to work.

Answer the following questions:
1.   Which of the two facilities described is more efficient?
2.   Which facility had the better charge efficiency (charge/change in function) and length-of-stay efficiency (ie, change in function/length of stay)?

CHECK YOUR RESPONSES

1.   a. Patient:
   - The patient is now unable to carry out his full duties
   - He is unhappy with his modified job duties
   - He wants to be able to return to his prior level of activities both at home and at work
   - He may feel accused of malingering, but then again maybe it would not be so bad to retire early on disability

   b. Physical therapist:
   - Wants "light duty" at work to remain only as a transition phase to full duty at work
   - By restricting a patient to lifting only 15 pounds, the patient is labeled, and this may limit future employment possibilities
   - Gains in range of motion and strength only have meaning to the physical therapist and not to the payer

   c. Employer:
   - Is concerned about cost
   - Is required to create a position of employment for the "light duty" employee, and the employer's needs may not be met
   - Most of the time the employer loses money

   d. Payer:
   - Wants the patient to return to work with minimum (but sufficient) treatment
   - Is not concerned about level of employee function at work (ie, light duty)
   - Would prefer to settle the case and limit risk of future liability for the employee's medical costs

2.

Outcome	Facility A	Facility B
	Return to work	Return to work
Length of disability	8 weeks	6 weeks
Number of visits	10	7 to 8
Total cost	$400	$420
Change in function (FRS)	53	45
Charge/FRS change	$7.55	$9.33
FRS change/number of visits	5.3	6.4
FRS change/length of disability	6.6	7.5

   - Facility A is less expensive overall, with a total cost of $400. The charge/FRS change represents how much it costs for each increase in unit of function. This value is also known as charge efficiency. Facility A's charge efficiency is $7.55, which is $1.78 less than facility B's charge efficiency.

- On the other hand, facility B has better length-of-stay efficiency. Length-of-stay efficiency represents the average functional change that occurs at each visit. Facility B had a length-of-stay efficiency of 6.4. This is 21% higher than facility A's length-of-stay efficiency of 5.3, which is evident through the fact that Harrison had fewer visits and returned to work sooner.
- The FRS change/length of disability values were calculated to show another way to determine length-of-stay efficiency. Again, notice that facility B had a higher length-of-stay efficiency than facility A.
- In comparing the charge/visit, you can see that facility A was less expensive than facility B. Therefore, it would be natural to think that facility A was the more efficient facility. However, facility B has better length-of-stay efficiency because its patient still went back to work in less time and with fewer visits. Therefore, it is important to look at both charge efficiency and length-of-stay efficiency when analyzing outcomes.

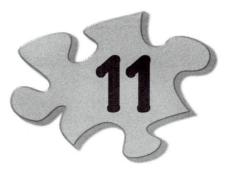

DOCUMENTATION REQUIREMENTS

Jenna Sawdon, MPT

I *magine yourself as a utilization reviewer for a health maintenance organization (HMO). You are a high school graduate and have 2 months of experience in the claims department. You took a self-directed medical terminology course 6 months ago, and your knowledge of anatomy is seemingly nonexistent. On your desk is the following request for further visits and reimbursement:*

Patient name: Richard Smith

Number of visits: 6

Diagnosis: (R) THR

   S: Feeling a little better

   O: Therapeutic exercise for (L) LE strengthening

   A: Doing well

   P: Continue with exercises as tolerated

Thank You,

Marvin Stevens, PT

Your job is to review the note and assess to what degree skilled physical therapy services have been provided. From the note, can you realistically gain an understanding of this patient's progress, functional gains, and rationale for physical therapy services? Subsequently, it is no surprise that you deny reim-

bursement for the past six visits and also deny further treatment. As you process the denial papers, you recognize the urgency with which physical therapists must modify their approach to the essential task of documentation.

VIEW OF DOCUMENTATION

Charting and documenting are habitually depicted as time-consuming, tedious, required tasks. Physical therapists view documentation as a "have to," so, therefore we just do it. However, each therapist's approach to documenting differs. Some spend vast amounts of time on explicitly detailed reports; some use such an array of unapproved abbreviations that fellow therapists have a difficult time deciphering the treatment intervention; some simply outline key aspects of an intervention. Moreover, we often fail to tailor our reports for those outside the profession who hold the purse strings for reimbursement of therapy services.[1]

As a consequence of numerous years of inconsistent and often inadequate documentation, payers of services have formed a potent and often unfavorable view about the physical therapy profession. Payers have questioned if physical therapists "ever get anyone well" and "why they need to do five things for each treatment."[1] Further complaints focus around "poor documentation of goals and progress, and poor objective data," and therapists "treat until death do us part."[1]

Such spirited negative reactions are serving as the driving force toward reform. With the shift to a managed care system, reports must clearly articulate to payers that physical therapy services are effective and efficient and that the outcome is worth the dollars spent.[1] To achieve this objective, therapists need to understand who reads our reports and what each group of readers wants.

READERS OF PHYSICAL THERAPY REPORTS

No matter what your style of documentation, your reports land in the hands of many people (Table 11.1).

Physical therapists must recognize that most individuals listed in Table 11.1 have never had any formalized training or inservices to assist them in understanding "what physical therapy is, what constitutes physical therapy expertise, how effective we are, what areas we evaluate, what different treatment approaches we utilize, the extent of our education, how autonomously we practice, what means we use to develop and monitor our treatment plans,

TABLE 11.1

COMMON READERS OF PHYSICAL THERAPY REPORTS

- Primary and referring physicians
- Physician's nursing staff
- Other physical therapists
- Occupational therapists
- Home health agencies
- Join Commission on Accreditation of Hospitals representatives
- Utilization review nurses
- Utilization review physicians
- Preferred provider organization staff
- Discharge planners
- Social services staff
- Workers' compensation claims adjusters
- Workers' compensation supervisors
- Preferred provider organization utilization review

- Group health claims auditors
- Medical bill review service staff
- Auditing firms
- Malpractice defense attorneys
- Malpractice plaintiff attorneys
- Jury members
- Physical therapist assistants
- Judges
- Expert witness for the defense
- Expert witness for the plaintiff
- HMO staff
- Medicare intermediary review nurses
- Medicare intermediary review therapists
- Utilization review team members
- Fraud investigators
- Multi-skilled health workers

Reprinted with permission from Stewart D, Abeln S, eds. Documenting Functional Outcomes in Physical Therapy. *St. Louis, Mo: Mosby-Year Book; 1993:38.*

and how efficient we are in obtaining patient recovery or return to function with different diagnoses."[1] Because many readers lack a medical background and hold little knowledge in general medical terminology and human anatomy, the need to change and/or modify our approach to documentation for third-party payers and other readers becomes even more apparent. It is not surprising that if the readers of our reports cannot follow or make sense of our notes, the likelihood for denial of reimbursement markedly increases.

IDEAL DOCUMENTATION FROM A PAYER'S PERSPECTIVE

The strongest tool we have to demonstrate our unique skill, expertise, and ability to make effective interventions with patients is our documentation. Our documentation must reflect what payers want to see. The repeatedly asked question is, "What do payers and other readers want in our reports?" Interviews with various payers provide us with applicable insight.

The optimal *initial report* from the payer's perspective entails[1]

- A clear statement of the problem(s) and why skilled physical therapy services are indicated—in terms understood by all readers and discussion of the effect on function
- Prior level of function

- A plan of action that directly addresses the problem(s), including a timeline for achieving the functional outcome
- The expected result in terms of function
- How long the treatment will take to achieve the expected result

The optimal *interim/progress report* entails[1]
- Restatement of the initial problem
- What you have done
- Why you have done it
- How the treatment has been effective in changing the initial problem and function
- How much longer you will have to treat the patient

The optimal *discharge report* entails[1]
- Restatement of the initial problem
- What you have done
- Why you have done it
- How it has been effective in changing the initial problem and function
- Whether there is a need for further services in a different environment (home program or gym maintenance program)

DOCUMENTATION AS A LEGAL RECORD

Tailoring our reports solely for reimbursement consideration is not enough. Documentation is also a legal record that displays a standard of care. Violations of the standard of patient care are often the driving force behind malpractice suits. Attorneys involved in medical malpractice cases customarily use the standard of care developed by the professional organization.[1] For physical therapy, the House of Delegates of the American Physical Therapy Association (APTA) developed the standards of care. Table 11.2 depicts an applicable portion from the APTA *Standards of Practice.*

The practice of physical therapy and documentation of the practice are both addressed in the *Standards of Practice.* Therefore, poor documentation constitutes patient negligence. So how can you protect yourself legally?

As part of your legal duty to each patient, you must provide accurate, complete, objective documentation of the patient's[1]
- Complaint(s)
- Relevant history
- Evaluative findings
- Informed consent for treatment

TABLE 11.2

STANDARDS OF PRACTICE

X. Informed Consent:
Physical therapist obtains the patient's informed consent in accordance with jurisdictional law before initiating physical therapy.

XI. Initial Evaluation:
Physical therapist performs and records an initial evaluation and interprets results to determine appropriate care for the individual.

XII. Plan of Care:
1. Physical therapist establishes and records a plan of care for the individual, based on the results of the evaluation.
2. Physical therapist involves the individual/significant other in the plan, implementation, and revision of the treatment program.
3. Physical therapist plans for discharge of the individual, taking into consideration goal achievement, and provides for appropriate follow-up referral.

XIII. Treatment:
1. Physical therapist provides or delegates and supervises the physical therapy treatment consistent with the results of the evaluation and plan of care.
2. Physical therapist records, on an ongoing basis, treatment rendered, progress, and change in status relative to the plan of care.

XIV. Re-evaluation:
Physical therapist reevaluates the individual and modifies the plan of care as indicated.

Reprinted from Standards of Practice. *Alexandria, Va: American Physical Therapy Association; 1990, with permission from the American Physical Therapy Association.*

Additional tactics to use when documenting or reporting that will serve as a strong defense include[1]

- Always writing on every line in the chart
- Writing with one pen
- Correcting mistakes by drawing a single line through the error and initialing (and dating, where required by law) the correction
- Do not edit prior entries except for correcting contemporaneous mistakes
- Do not backdate an omission in the treatment record
- Documenting any omitted prior entry as a new entry
- Writing legibly—print if necessary
- Do not express personal feelings about a patient (ie, "patient is a malingerer")
- Do not argue with or disparage other health care providers in the record
- Avoid including extraneous verbiage not related to treatment in the record
- Avoid using terms or abbreviations not universally understood by all providers treating the patient (listed in Appendix 1)

INCIDENT REPORTS

Incident reporting is a critical element in the documentation process. Collecting and recording the information of an adverse incident can protect you and aid in the management of your risks as a practitioner. While each physical therapy setting differs slightly in documenting unfavorable incidents, certain universal rules predominate.

An incident report includes[1]

- Identity of the patient
- Complete description of the incident in objective terms
- Where the incident occurred
- When the incident occurred
- Circumstances surrounding the incident
- All potential witnesses to the incident
- Any equipment the patient may have been using or working with at the time of the incident (name the manufacturer of the equipment)
- Actions taken to mitigate the injuries sustained by the patient as a result of the incident
- All comments the patient may have made regarding the incident
- Whether the patient may have somehow contributed to the injury

Because incident reports are confidential, no incident should be considered too minor to report.[1-4] However, health care providers are often uncertain about when to generate an incident report. The following case example serves to illustrate an unfortunate, yet pragmatic, situation physical therapists encounter.

> *Art, an outpatient with a diagnosis of low back pain, arrives at the physical therapy clinic for his fourth treatment. As you, therapist X, enter the treatment room to apply a moist heat pack, you notice a patch of red and blistered skin extending roughly 2 inches on either side of Art's L4 - S1 spinous processes. You inquire about the injured area, and Art states that during his treatment 2 days ago, the hot pack was left on for too long. Upon arriving home, Art reports that the skin on his back was "burning" and "felt raw." While changing his shirt, Art looked in a mirror and noticed the burn on his low back.*

Because therapist X is the one who observed Art's condition and heard Art's statements about potential cause, it is the responsibility of therapist X to write the incident report. In the report, therapist X needs to objectively and concisely document what was seen and heard. The following entry describing the event would be appropriate.

Art arrived for treatment of moist heat and exercise at 0830 hours, February 15, 1998. While Art was getting on the treatment table, I noticed a 2-inch round blister, extending from both sides of his L4-S1 spinous processes. The skin surrounding the blister was erythematous, and the wound was dry. Art stated to me, "The hot pack was left on too long during my last treatment, and I got burned." I withheld application of the hot pack and contacted Dr. L in the acute care clinic, who agreed to evaluate Art later in the morning. Follow-up pending.

While the illustrated entry above is an appropriate means of documenting an incident, facility-generated incident report forms are also used (Table 11.3).

PREVIOUS DOCUMENTATION MODEL

Although reporting forms vary, the majority are based on the subjective, objective, assessment plan (SOAP) format. This format has met most of the primary requirements for successful documentation over the years.[2] However, the SOAP note format has its inherent problems. According to Swanson,[3] this style of reporting contains a built-in bias because it assumes that improvement in physical capabilities leads directly to improved function.

To avoid this bias and report in a manner that explicitly demonstrates functional assessment and outcome, a new approach is needed. Two such proposed methods attempt to meet this objective. Both methods are predicated on functional limitations.

Modifying the SOAP Note

Because the SOAP note is easy to use and familiar to many, it is logical to modify this format to make it more easily understood by those outside the profession. To accomplish this transformation, Abeln calls for three changes to the current pattern of SOAP reporting.[4]

- Modify the "objective" section: This section typically lists impairments (range of motion measurements, manual muscle testing grades, girth measurements, and gait patterns) and neglects to detail the objective functional limitations.
- Impairment versus disability: Before proceeding further, we need to clear up the often troublesome terms *impairment* and *disability*. As defined by the World Health Organization, *impairment* is any loss or abnormality of psychologic, physiologic, or anatomic structure or function (range of motion limitations, strength of muscle performance, edema) and *disability* is any restriction or lack of ability to perform an activity of daily living (inability to perform self-grooming, ie, bathing,

TABLE 11.3

EXAMPLE OF AN INCIDENT REPORT

Quality Assurance Risk Management Report

WARNING: The information contained in this quality assurance document is confidential and subject to privilege under applicable state and federal law. Penalties may apply for unauthorized release. Do not file or refer to this document in any treatment record.

1. Date/time/location of incident: _____
2. Name/age/gender of person(s) involved: _____
3. If incident involved a patient, state patient's principal diagnosis and name(s) of attending physician(s): _____
4. Description of event: _____
5. Condition of patient and/or other persons affected, after occurrence:
6. Name(s), address(es), phone number(s) of witness(es), if any, and each witness's description of event: _____
7. Brief description of treatment rendered, if any: _____
8. Name, title, and position of person completing form: _____
9. Signature of preparer and date of report: _____

Note to preparer of report: Forward through department or service chief to facility risk manager within 24 hours. Notify risk manager telephonically of event immediately after emergency, if any, is resolved.

Reprinted with permission from Scott RW. Adverse incidents, abandonment, and other special circumstances. In: Scott RW. Legal Aspects of Documenting Patient Care, as well as © 1994 Aspen Publishers, Inc.

dressing). It is imperative that we link the impairment to the patient's disability status because claims denial is often due to failure to connect the two terms.[4]

- Modify the "assessment" section: Along with the normally included treatment goals and the often mentioned general assessment of the patient's status (ie, "tol, treatment well"), a brief listing of therapy problems is called for. You should only list those problems that can be improved through therapeutic intervention and, subsequently, will improve the patient's function. Also added to this section is a list of "complication" factors to therapy.[4] Included in this list are other factors that may limit the patient's function, (ie, clinical depression, outstanding litigation, or lack of social support system).[4]
- Modify treatment goals: We must change the emphasis of a therapeutic intervention from improvement of impairments to improvement of function.

An example of the proposed changes are depicted in Table 11.4.

TABLE 11.4

EVALUATION REVISED TO IMPROVE REPORTING OF FUNCTION

S:
Pt. is a 42-year-old male carpenter who injured his L knee two weeks ago playing football. Five days ago, he underwent a L medial meniscectomy. He has been walking as much as he can since outpatient surgery and was referred to PT to increase ROM and strengthen L leg. Pt. states that he currently is working 4 hours a day as a result of the injury/surgery and is working in a modified capacity (completing bid paperwork) because he can no longer do the frequent walking and stair and ladder climbing that are essential elements of his job.
Therapy Problems: Loss of joint motion, tissue inflammation, weakness, difficulty coordinating gait cycle to reduce knee stress.
Complicating Factors: Outstanding litigation against recreation leader.
O:
Impairments: ROM: RLE-WNL for hip, knee, and ankle; LLE-ankle-WNL; knee -80 * active flex/87 * passive flex (norm 120+); -20 * active ext in sit/-14 * passive ext in sit.
Strength: Manual muscle test. RLE-WNL; LLE-ankle and hip WNL; knee-quadriceps 3-/5; hamstrings 4/5.
Swelling: L knee red and tender to palpation along scar line; R knee 6 inches above knee=19 inches; mid-joint=16 inches; 6 inches below knee=17 inches; L knee 6 inches above knee=20 inches; mid-joint=19 inches; 6 inches below knee=18 inches.
Gait: Minimal stance time L, poor swing phase.
Pain: Pt. pain on 10-point visual analog scale prior to activity 5/10; after ambulating 100 feet 8.5/10.
Traditional Goals Related to Impairment: Increase ROM, decrease pain, increase strength.
Functional Goals

Activity	Performance	Due date
Standing balance	Indep w/o device 10 ft.	in 4 visits
Flat terrain ambulation	indep w/o device 100 ft.	in 6 visits
Unassisted walking uneven terrain	Tolerate for 30 min 5x/day	in 6 visits
Ascend & descend unassisted	Tolerate for 20 min 3x/day	in 7 visits
Ascend & descend ladder	2x/day	

Functional Limitations

Activity	Current status
Sit-stand transfer	Independent
Standing balance	Performs independently with partial weight bearing and two crutches; without crutches, unable to maintain balance > 1 min
Flat terrain ambulation	Performs with two axillary crutches, takes 25 sec for 20 ft. and tolerates < 6 min
Uneven terrain ambulation	Unable to maintain balance over rough terrain
Stair climbing	Able to ascend 2 steps only using crutches and rail (speed 1 min); descends two steps with crutches (speed 30 sec)
Ladder climbing	Unable to perform

A:
Medical diagnosis status post menisectomy is further defined to include residual L knee inflammation
Therapy Problems: Loss of joint motion, tissue inflammation, weakness, difficulty coordinating gait cycle to reduce knee stress
Complicating Factors: Outstanding litigation against recreation league
P:
Lower extremity strength and ROM training (home exercise and Biodex), anti-inflammatory modalities, and education in independent pain control

Reprinted from Abeln S. Improving functional reporting. PT-Magazine of Physical Therapy. 1996; 4(3)26-30, with permission from the American Physical Therapy Association.

TABLE 11.5

Six Steps in the
Functional Outcome Report (FOR) Model

Step	Clinical reasoning process	FOR report item
1.	Establish patient need	Report reason for referral
2.	Analyze patient performance	Identify and report functional limitation
3.	Identify clinician impression	Establish physical therapy assessment
4.	Postulate relationships between impairment and performance	Identify therapy problems
5.	Predict functional outcome	List functional outcome goals
6.	Devise treatment strategy	Present treatment plan and rationale

Reprinted with permission from Swanson G. Functional outcome reporting. In: Stewart D, Abeln S, eds. Documenting Functional Outcomes in Physical Therapy. *St. Louis, Mo: Mosby-Year Book;1993:107.*

Shift to Functional Outcome Reporting

Similar to the previously mentioned modified SOAP note format, the functional outcome report enables therapists to use their clinical reasoning and document the functional aftermath of a disorder.

As defined by Blue Cross of California, to be considered a functional outcome, patient status after therapy must meet three criteria.[3]

1. Meaningful outcome is one in which the activity level achieved by the patient as a result of physical therapy is that level necessary for the patient to function most effectively at home or at work.
2. Practical outcome represents the most economical and efficient method by which to perform the desired activity.
3. Sustained outcome demonstrates that the activity level achieved is maintained outside the clinical environment and over a period of time.

According to Swanson, there are six steps in the Functional Outcome Report Model (Table 11.5).

DOCUMENTING FOR MEDICARE

For a patient to be covered under Medicare Part A (hospital, home health care, inpatient skilled nursing facility) or Part B (outpatient), two criteria must be met. The services must:[5]

TABLE 11.6

EFFECT OF THE CRITERIA FOR REASONABLE AND NECESSARY SERVICE ON DOCUMENTATION

Criteria	Questions documentation must answer
1. Services are based on accepted standard that is specific and effective for the condition	Is service documented accepted treatment based on condition?
2. Service is at the level of complexity or patient's condition requires that a physical therapist perform the services in order for it to be safely and effectively rendered	Does the service require the judgment, knowledge, and skill of the physical therapist or could ancillary personnel do it?
3. Expectation that the outcome will occur or physical therapist's skill is required to establish a safe and effective maintenance program based on disease state	Is there demonstration that a functional or measurable gain has occurred? Are the therapist's skills required to develop a maintenance program?
4. Amount, frequency, and duration are reasonable	Is there a strong indication that the patient's condition supports the frequency, intensity, and duration of treatment?

Reprinted with permission from Esposto L. Applying functional outcome assessment to Medicare documentation. In: Stewart D, Abeln S, eds. Documenting Functional Outcomes in Physical Therapy. *St. Louis, Mo: Mosby-Year Book; 1993:141.*

1. Relate directly and specifically to an active written treatment program established by a physician or a physical therapist providing the services
2. Be reasonable and necessary to the treatment of an individual illness or injury

As stated in the Medicare guidelines, four conditions classify what is reasonable and necessary. To write in such a manner that meets the four conditions, you should be able to answer the questions depicted in Table 11.6.[3]

ELEMENTS OF MEDICARE DOCUMENTATION

Elements of Medicare documentation include an evaluation, a monthly summary, and a discharge summary.

Initial Evaluation

Three major elements of documentation are necessary to justify the need for physical therapy intervention and to assess the rehabilitation potential of the patient.[5]

1.   Justification for referral:
   - Reason for referral
   - Pertinent medical history of current medical problem
   - Previous level of function
   - The need for a physical therapist to perform the procedure
2.   Assessment of findings (in objective and specific terms):
   - Range of motion
   - Strength
   - Pain
   - Gait
   - Prior level of function

To determine functional levels:
   - Transfers/bed mobility
   - Balance
   - Posture
   - Ambulation
   - Level of independence with activities of daily living
   - Chronic conditions
   - Efficiency
3.   Treatment plan and goals:
   - List therapy modalities
   - Frequency and duration of treatment
   - Provide an estimated time line for care

Monthly Summary

The monthly summary must include the following:

1.   Justify why physical therapy is indicated. State the diagnosis and/or reason for the referral or continuing care.
2.   Justify why the patient was treated throughout the claim period. State the patient's progress in objective and measurable terms.

TABLE 11.7

ESSENTIAL ELEMENTS OF A
MEDICARE DISCHARGE SUMMARY

Diagnosis/reason for referral	Why therapy?
Objective data: State overall impairment and function from the date of initial evaluation and last billing period to justify current and total billing period	Why therapy continued?
Plan of care that takes into consideration need for future services. State only goals met in your facility and that there is a need for further services at a less intense level or in a different environment. If not appropriate, state what, if anything, the patient should continue to do on a home program or maintenance program	Why discharged?

Reprinted with permission from Esposto L. Applying functional outcome assessment to Medicare documentation. In: Stewart D, Abeln S, eds. Documenting Functional Outcomes in Physical Therapy. *St. Louis, Mo: Mosby-Year Book; 1993:157.*

---

3. Justify why treatment should be continued. State the unmet goals and how you will progress the patient to attain these goals.

Discharge Summary

The discharge summary must be written when a patient is discharged to another setting or when therapy is terminated. Table 11.7 describes the essential elements of a Medicare discharge summary.

According to several Medicare consultants to Blue Cross of California, "the reviewer is looking for complete records, demonstration of the need for skilled physical therapy, and sound clinical judgment in terms of patient treatment, case management, and outcome."[6] Five common reasons for Medicare denial for reimbursement include the following:

1. Lack of, or need for, skilled physical therapy. According to Medicare, treatment can safely and effectively be performed only by a registered physical therapist or under his or her supervision.
2. No significant improvement within a reasonable and predictable amount of time.

- Repetitive service
- Insignificant improvement or plateau in progress
- Inability to sustain goals
- No overall improvement
3. Routine multiple rechecks.
4. Routine screening evaluations.
5. Duplication of services. If a single service (physical therapist, occupational therapist, registered nurse) could provide the care, only one service will be covered.

It is important to remember that documentation encompasses all aspects of patient management. Along with treatment interventions, documentation of patient care conferences, communications (telephone, fax, computer, etc), coordination of care with family members/caregivers and other health care professionals, record reviews, and discharge planning all need to be included in a patient's chart.[7]

In the past 5 years, computerized record-keeping has been gaining recognition and application. One example is *PT Homecare Doc*, a documentation product for physical therapists, which is being used in home health care throughout the United States and in seven foreign countries. This form of documentation has been estimated to save therapists up to 75% of the time normally spent on handwritten notes.

Because non-reimbursement decisions made by payers or utilization review companies are often done on the basis of inadequate documentation, it is clearly time to improve our reporting skills.[2] According to Abeln, "we must accept reporting skills as an essential part of our practice and recognize that, although our patients may find our interventions invaluable, it is only through our reports that utilization reviewers, claims adjusters, lawyers, managed care companies, physicians, and case managers can judge the effectiveness of our interventions."[4]

SUMMARY

In today's dynamic heath care environment, it is crucial to change/modify our reporting style. We must know who will be reading our documentation and what each reader is looking for in an initial report, interim report, and discharge summary. We must recognize that our reports also serve as legal records, displaying a standard of patient care. Incident reporting is another integral element of documentation. Each therapist must be aware of the essential information that must be reported following an adverse incident. Strategies such as writing on every line in the chart, writing with one pen, and correcting mistakes with a single drawn line through the error will serve as a strong defense when documenting and can protect you legally.

The use of the SOAP note format contains a built-in bias because it assumes that improvement in physical capabilities leads directly to improved function. Two new methods of reporting were introduced that avoid this bias. The first method involves modifying the SOAP note's objective and assessment sections and proposes a shift from improvement of impairments to improvement of function and the relationship between the two. The second method incorporates a shift to functional outcome reporting. To use the Functional Outcome Report model, there are six steps in the process.

Documenting for Medicare needs not create as many headaches and additional paperwork if each therapist comprehends the definition of "reasonable and necessary," knows how to write in a style that meets the conditions of "reasonable and necessary," and understands the components to report in an initial evaluation, monthly report, and discharge summary. Understanding reasons for Medicare noncoverage and modifying your reporting will improve your rate of Medicare reimbursement.

Physical therapy documentation is not for the sole purpose of reimbursement and/or further authorization. Another critical function of documentation is that it serves as our memory and guidance system.[6] "It establishes what our patient's goals are, what we intend to do to meet them, and what the patient's response is to treatment. We use this system to help us make clinical decisions as to whether our treatment approach is appropriate and effective."[6]

REFERENCES

1. Abeln S. Importance of documentation to patient care reimbursement. In: Stewart D, Abeln S, eds. *Documenting Functional Outcomes in Physical Therapy*. St. Louis, Mo: Mosby-Year Book Inc; 1993.
2. Clifton D. "Tolerated treatment well" may no longer be tolerated. *PT-Magazine of Physical Therapy*. 1995; 3(10);24,26-27.
3. Swanson G. Functional outcome reporting. In: Stewart D, Abeln S, eds. *Documenting Functional Outcomes in Physical Therapy*. St. Louis, Mo: Mosby-Year Book Inc; 1993.
4. Abeln S. Utilization Review-Improving functional reporting. *PT-Magazine of Physical Therapy*. 1996;4(3):26,28-30.
5. Esposto L. Applying functional outcome assessment to Medicare documentation. In: Stewart D, Abeln S, eds. *Documenting Functional Outcomes in Physical Therapy*. St. Louis, Mo: Mosby-Year Book Inc; 1993.
6. Bernstein F, Eguchi K, Messer S, et al.Insurance reimbursement and the physical therapist-Documentation for outpatient physical therapy. *Clinical Management in Physical Therapy*. 1987;7(2):28-33.
7. Appendix II. Code of ethics and guide for professional conduct. *Phys Ther*. 1995;75:740-762.

TEST YOUR SKILLS

1. Name five potential readers of your documentation.
2. From the payer's perspective:
   - What should the initial report include?
   - What should the interim/progress report include?
   - What should the discharge report include?
3. What must you document as part of your legal duty to each patient?
4. Name five strategies for documenting that can serve as a strong defense?
5. What is included in an incident report?
6. What three changes are proposed that will modify the SOAP note to avoid its built-in bias?
7. Distinguish between an impairment and a disability. Give an example of each.
8. According to Blue Cross of California, what three criteria must be met in order to be considered a functional outcome?
9. Name the six steps in the Functional Outcome Reporting model.
10. According to Medicare guidelines, what four conditions define "reasonable and necessary"?
11. Name the major elements in
    - An initial Medicare evaluation
    - A Medicare monthly summary
    - A Medicare discharge summary

CHECK YOUR RESPONSES

1. Any five of the following would be appropriate:
    *   Primary and referring physicians
    *   Group health claims auditors
    *   Physician's nursing staff
    *   Medical bill review service staff
    *   Other physical therapists
    *   Auditing firms
    *   Occupational therapists
    *   Malpractice defense attorneys
    *   Home health agencies
    *   Malpractice plaintiff attorneys
    *   JCAHO representatives
    *   Jury members
    *   Utilization review nurses
    *   Judges
    *   Utilization review physicians
    *   Expert witness for the defense
    *   Preferred provider organization staff
    *   Expert witness for the plaintiff
    *   Discharge planners
    *   HMO staff
    *   Social services staff
    *   Medicare intermediary review nurses
    *   Workers' compensation claims adjusters
    *   Medicare intermediary review therapists
    *   Utilization review team members
    *   Workers' compensation supervisors
    *   Fraud investigators
    *   Preferred provider organization utilization review
    *   Multi-skilled health workers
    *   Physical therapist assistants

2. The optimal *initial report* from the payer's perspective entails:
    *   A clear statement of the problem(s) and why skilled physical therapy services are indicated—in terms understood by all readers and discussion of the effect on function

- Prior level of function
- A plan of action that directly addresses the problem(s), including a time line for achieving the functional outcome
- The expected result in terms of function
- How long the treatment will take to achieve the expected result

The optimal *interim/progress report* entails:
- Restatement of the initial problem
- What you have done
- Why you have done it
- How the treatment has been effective in changing the initial problem and function
- How much longer you will have to treat the patient

The optimal *discharge report* entails:
- Restatement of initial problem
- What you have done
- Why you have done it
- How it has been effective in changing the initial problem and function
- Whether there is a need for further services in a different environment (ie, home program or gym maintenance program)

3. As part of your legal duty to each patient, you must provide accurate, complete, objective documentation of the patient's
- Complaint(s)
- Relevant history
- Evaluative findings
- Informed consent for treatment

4. Tactics to use when documenting or reporting that will serve as a strong defense include:
- Always write on every line in the chart
- Write with one pen
- Correct mistakes by drawing a single line through the error and initialing (and dating, where required by law) the correction
- Do not edit prior entries except for correcting contemporaneous mistakes
- Do not backdate an omission in the treatment record
- Document any omitted prior entry as a new entry
- Write legibly—print if necessary
- Do not express personal feelings about a patient (eg, "patient is a malingerer")

- Do not argue with or disparage other health care providers in the record
- Avoid including extraneous verbiage not related to treatment in the record
- Avoid using terms or abbreviations not universally understood by all providers treating the patient

5. An *incident report* includes:
   - Identity of the patient
   - Complete description of the incident in objective terms
   - Where the incident occurred
   - When the incident occurred
   - Circumstances surrounding the incident
   - All potential witnesses to the incident
   - Any equipment the patient may have been using or working with at the time of the incident. Name the manufacturer of the equipment.
   - Actions taken to mitigate the injuries sustained by the patient as a result of the incident
   - all comments the patient may have made regarding the incident
   - Whether the patient may have somehow contributed to the injury

6. Modify the objective section:
   This section typically lists impairments (range of motion measurements, manual muscle testing grades, girth measurements, and gait patterns) and neglects to detail the objective functional limitations.

   Modify the assessment section:
   Along with the normally included treatment goals and the often mentioned general assessment of the patient's status (ie, "tol, treatment well"), a brief listing of therapy problems is called for. You should only list those problems that can be improved through therapeutic intervention and, subsequently, will improve the patient's function. Also added to this section is a list of "complication" factors to therapy. Included in this list are other factors that may limit the patient's function, (ie, clinical depression, outstanding litigation, or lack of social support system).

   Modify the treatment goals:
   We must change the emphasis of a therapeutic intervention from improvement of impairments to improvement of function.

7. Impairment: Any loss or abnormality of psychologic, physiologic, or anatomic structure or function (examples may include range of motion limitations, strength of muscle performance, edema)

Disability: Any restriction or lack of ability to perform an activity of daily living (examples may include inability to perform self-grooming, like bathing, dressing)

8. Three criteria for functional outcome:
   - *Meaningful outcome* is one in which the activity level achieved by the patient as a result of physical therapy is that level necessary for the patient to function most effectively at home or at work.
   - *Practical outcome* represents the most economical and efficient method by which to perform the desired activity.
   - *Sustained outcome* demonstrates that the activity level achieved is maintained outside the clinical environment and over a period of time.

9.

Step	Clinical reasoning process	FOR report item
1.	Establish patient need	Report reason for referral
2.	Analyze patient performance	Identify and report functional limitation
3.	Identify clinician impression	Establish physical therapy assessment
4.	Postulate relationships between impairment and performance	Identify therapy problems
5.	Predict functional outcome	List functional outcome goals
6.	Devise treatment strategy	Present treatment plan and rationale

10. Services are based on accepted standard that is *specific* and *effective* for the condition. Service is at the level of complexity or patient's condition requiring a physical therapist perform the services in order for it to be safely and effectively rendered. Expectation that the outcome will occur or a physical therapist's skill is required to establish a safe and effective maintenance program based on disease state. Amount, frequency, and duration are reasonable.

11. Initial evaluation: three major elements of documentation are necessary to justify the need for physical therapy intervention and to assess the rehabilitation potential of the patient.

    Justification for referral:
    - Reason for referral
    - Pertinent medical history of current medical problem

- Previous level of function
- The need for a physical therapist to perform the procedure

Assessment of findings—in objective and specific terms, list:
- Range of motion
- Strength
- Pain
- Gait
- Prior level of function

To determine functional levels:
- Transfers/bed mobility
- Balance
- Posture
- Ambulation
- Level of independence with activities of daily living
- Chronic conditions
- Efficiency

Treatment plan and goals:
- List therapy modalities
- Frequency and duration of treatment
- Provide an estimated time-line for care

Monthly summary must:
- Justify why physical therapy is indicated
- State the diagnosis and/or reason for the referral or continuing care
- Justify why the patient was treated throughout the claim period
- State the patient's progress in objective and measurable terms
- Justify why treatment should be continued
- State the unmet goals and how you will progress the patient to attain these goals

Discharge summary must be written when a patient is discharged to another setting or when therapy is terminated. The following describes the essential elements of a Medicare discharge summary.

1. Diagnosis/reason for referral:
- Why therapy?
2. Objective data:
- Why therapy is continued?
- State overall impairment and function from the date of initial evaluation and last billing period to justify current and total billing period.
3. Plan of care that takes into consideration need for future services.
4. Why discharged?

- State only goals met in your facility and that there is a need for further services at a less intense level or in a different environment.
- If not appropriate, state what, if anything, the patient should continue to do on a home program or maintenance program.

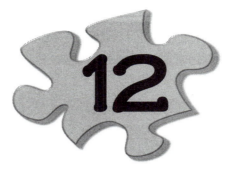

UTILIZATION MANAGEMENT

Noelle Righter-Freer, MPT

Mr. Wilkinson is no stranger to the hydro-therapy unit at Anderson Outpatient Center. He has been treated for a malleolar ulcer for the past year. His physical therapist, known to provide the best wound care in town, has provided consistent treatment. He has faithfully guided the slow improvement of the wound, sticking close to the referring physician's orders to address the healing plateaus. Mr. Wilkinson's therapist tells him that he should be grateful that he has Medicare insurance to rely on, as other means of insurance may have dropped him long ago based on his multiple risk factors. His therapist, engulfed in his busy schedule, fails to file his monthly summary on time. Upon sending in the update, he finds that Mr. Wilkinson's wound treatment has been denied for the past year on the basis of "lack of progress." This family-owned practice will not be reimbursed for the hours of treatment or supplies.

This case scenario is based on an actual account. Wilkinson's therapist will have to write off this year of treatment as pro-bono service. Had someone been reviewing this patient's chart regularly, he or she may have been aware of Medicare restrictions to prevent this revenue loss. Utilization management (UM), in this case, would have greatly benefited this family-owned practice.

The information in this chapter is designed to equip you with knowledge about UM so that you may prevent and combat potentially harmful occurrences similar to the one described on Page 209.

UTILIZATION MANAGEMENT

UM, much like its predecessor, utilization review (UR), is defined as the monitoring of provider performance in comparison to a standard or expectation. *Utilization management* is a response to finding variable clinical practice patterns for the same clinical condition. This variation in practice is believed to cause unnecessary care and therefore a cost burden to society."[1] In other words, it can be thought of as a "watch dog" or as a means of holding practitioners accountable to necessary and quality treatment. Reviewed case by case, it ensures that each patient qualifies for the level of care he or she is receiving through prevention of prolonged lengths of stay, excessive number of visits, and unnecessary treatment.

Also defined as "a management technique used to review a prescribed course of medical care," it can serve two primary purposes:
- To improve the quality of care by deterring unnecessary or inappropriate treatment
- To save money by imposing cost-containment strategies[2]

UM may or may not indirectly affect reimbursement for treatment. Like the managed care environment, UM is ever-changing, which makes it difficult to define with concrete, clear parameters.

LIFE WITHOUT UM OR UR

Before 1965, there was no UR. Health care consumers became increasingly concerned about the quality of their treatment, and health care costs were determined predominantly by health care providers. Consequently, the potential for fraud and abuse was greater, as no one was appointed to regulate health care with questionable quality, necessity, or duration.

When Medicare and Medicaid first came into existence, the Health Care Financing Administration required that a UR process be implemented.[3] Other programs then began to follow in the footsteps of government programs to ensure quality and medical necessity of treatment. In the 1970s, the Joint Commission on Accreditation of Healthcare Organizations began to require defined standards of UR in hospital and medical review.

From 1980 to 1992, health care costs rose from 9% to 14% of the nation's gross domestic product.[4] The need for a review system became even more urgent as a means to monitor for price control and reduce unnecessary or unreasonable expenditures.

Today, UR exists (many say in excess), in professional associations and governmental and accrediting agencies. It sometimes takes on an ambiguous form, as the criteria and regulations vary broadly across the spectrum. Many health care organizations claim to theoretically have a UR system; however, it often becomes a low priority as it falls through the cracks of paperwork and time constraints.

Without a strong institutional or organizational commitment, UR is often conducted haphazardly, and providers are held accountable solely by retrospective reimbursement. Here, the payer decides not to reimburse "inappropriate" treatment "after the fact."

Most recently, a shift is being made to UM, in which, ideally, inappropriate treatment is regulated in progress.

COMMON QUESTIONS ASKED BY PHYSICAL THERAPISTS ABOUT UR

What is the Difference Between UR and UM?

The main difference between UR and UM is that UR is a retrospective review, while UM is a prospective review. Today's trend is moving toward UM's prospective processes. UM "involves the prospective management of medical cases to assure that only medically necessary, reasonable, and appropriate services are provided from a reimbursement standpoint."[5]

UM can prevent inappropriate care from continuing, while care is deemed inappropriate "after the fact" by UR.[6] For a more in-depth look at the differences, see Table 12.1.

Anderson Outpatient Center, mentioned at the beginning of the chapter, could have benefited from UM. "Excessive" treatments could have been monitored and prevented if they were deemed inappropriate or exceeded the allotted number of visits.

So What Exactly is Medically Necessary and Reasonable?

Medical necessity is defined as "treatment that is essential, appropriate, and effective."[7] To remain within the confines of this definition, you must be familiar with the words in this UR glossary:

TABLE 12.1

COMPARISON OF UTILIZATION REVIEW AND UTILIZATION MANAGEMENT

Utilization review	Utilization management
Primarily retrospective review	Primarily prospective review
May lead to provider profiling	Includes provider profiling
Makes no attempt to direct care	Deliberately attempts to direct care
Does not involve case management	Involves case management
Identifies "acceptable care"	Identifies "optimal outcomes"

Reprinted from Clifton DW. A shift toward utilization management. PT-Magazine of Physical Therapy. 1995;3(6):32-35, with permission from the American Physical Therapy Association.

- Essential treatment—treatment required to return a patient to his or her pre-morbid level of function or to prevent further deterioration.[7]
- Appropriate treatment—consistent with the nature and severity of the patients' condition.[7]
- Effective treatment—consistent with the best available scientific evidence of efficacy.[7]

The Florida Workers' Compensation Law sheds a bit more light on the subject by describing *medically necessary and reasonable* as

> *...Any service or supply used to identify or treat illness or injury which is appropriate to the patient's diagnosis, consistent with the location of the service, and with the level of care provided. The service should be widely accepted by the practicing peer group, should be based on scientific criteria, and should be reasonably safe. The service may not be of an experimental, investigative, or research nature.*[6]

How is UR Conducted and Regulated?

That depends on whether UR is internal or external review. *Internal review* focuses more on quality and appropriateness of care delivered by evaluating indicators in chart documentation that reflect necessity and timeliness of services provided. This type of review ensures that the organization will be reimbursed, reduces treatment risks, and pinpoints system problems. This is usually conducted by a staff member who is in a full-time position in the health care institution or organization to review charts. This position is required for institutional accreditation. The reviewer is usually a health professional, often a registered nurse.

In acute, sub-acute, and rehabilitation settings, internal UR may be conducted weekly in the form of team conference meetings. In these meetings, the

UR health professional consults with the in-house patients' skilled care providers to determine whether the patients are appropriate to remain in-house for skilled treatment. The team of providers present for recommendations may consist of nurses, physicians, occupational, speech, respiratory, or physical therapists.

During *external review*, the reviewer is not an employee of the organization, but an outsider who objectively reviews charts of multiple departments. External review focuses on appropriateness of care to determine reimbursement. Reviewers ensure that patient documentation reflects regional and state standards of practice and falls within reimbursement contract limits. Most likely, this person will be a nurse or clerical worker; few are physical therapists.[7]

Reviewers operate on one of three different levels of review.[8] Each individual involved in the review process has a different level of clinical knowledge and understanding of physical therapy. As the levels increase in number, so does the power of decision making and regulation.

- Level one—typically non-medical personnel with limited training in medical terminology and a limited understanding of rehabilitation.
- Level two—typically medical personnel (nurse, vocational counselor).
- Level three—peer review done by the medical director of the plan. A physical therapist is often involved at this level. This is an example of "like reviewing like."[2]

Does UR Determine Whether or Not I Get Reimbursed?

Generally, UR is not the sole factor determining reimbursement. Theoretically, UR is conducted more as a quality management system that catches unnecessary treatment in progress and stops it before the provider is denied reimbursement. Fiduciary responsibilities instead lie with the payer through a process like *claims review*. This review process, which affects reimbursement, is often confused with UR.

Claims review is "primarily an internal insurance or payer function that examines claims eligibility, policy coverage and limitations, and other administrative issues."[2] Many fiduciary companies hire UR companies to screen cases before they are passed on to claims review. Criteria for claims review often closely parallel UR criteria. In this arrangement, the cases that do not pass the UR criteria, of course, are denied reimbursement or certification by claims review.

Where Does Peer Review Fit into the Scene?

Peer review is a term often used interchangeably with UR. Although the two share characteristics, they are not entirely the same.

Peer review is, by definition, "a voluntary system by which individuals of similar background assess the quality of services provided by those of the same professional background" and as "a process that examines and evaluates the standards of care among staff members of similar levels of experience."[2]

While UR focuses on cost effectiveness and appropriateness of service, peer review assesses according to practice standards, ethical codes, timeliness, frequency, duration, outcome of treatment interventions, and appropriateness. *Internal peer review* is usually involved with an institution's quality improvement (QI) system (see Chapter 14) more so than for reimbursement purposes. Documents developed by the American Physical Therapy Association (APTA) to help guide you through the peer review process are available through the APTA Service Center—(800) 999-2782 ext. 3395.

How Are UR Criteria Developed?

Criteria vary across the spectrum, depending upon the originators. Some of the more predominant criteria may originate from independent UR agencies, known as utilization review organizations (UROs), or Medicare's peer review organizations.[3] The latter are comprised of groups of physicians. Often criteria are written by UROs used in UR agencies such as the Utilization Review Accreditation Commission.[9]

Many hospitals are developing baselines for critical pathways and treatment protocols to decide treatment norms. *Critical pathways* are defined as "optimal sequencing and timing of interventions developed by a multidisciplinary team for a particular diagnosis."[10] These methods pinpoint what patient outcomes vary from the established standards. These are often recorded on an institution's software database. This information is compared to similar patients' diagnoses during their stays. Once a patient's treatment variance is recognized, providers and reviewers can decide if the variance is appropriate. They may analyze what, if anything, went wrong and can then decide what can be done in the future to correct it. An example of a critical pathway for a total knee replacement is illustrated in Appendix 8.

These criteria may take the form of review criteria or practice guidelines through retrospective statistics. These statistics follow the 80/20 rule, which states "80% of the cases that involve a given diagnosis will pass the UR screen, whereas 20% of the cases will be subject to further scrutiny."[11] Criteria such as length of stay and costs are examined by central tendency measures, with a bell-shaped curve along with the 80/20 rule to determine inappropriate variances. Medicare's effort to standardize this data collection is in the form of uniform clinical data sets (UCDs). UCDs analyze patterns of procedure utilization and outcomes that are tailored to specific patient populations.[3]

Do These Review Systems Help or Hinder Physical Therapy Service?

Much controversy enters when this question arises. Many practitioners complain that their autonomy and creativity are stifled when their documentation is constantly reviewed by others and the extra paperwork required is time consuming. Other practitioners argue that if the provider's clinical decisions are sharpened, skills are polished, and documentation is accurate, UR will not get in the way of quality treatment.[12] However, many believe it is important to remember what health care would be like without a review system.

Like it or not, UR is certain to grow with payers' needs for validation of quality and providers' needs for independent review to keep in compliance with the mechanisms of payer scrutiny.[1]

Here lies room for managers and/or supervisors to be innovative and design a "low maintenance" UR paperwork system. Data entry and tabulation by computer are optimal time-efficient systems offered today. Payers and UR reviewers who document activity and claim status on electronic systems allow clinicians easy access to communicate and keep current on information via computer. This type of system reduces delays caused by phone calls, faxes, and availability for human communication.

Why Should Physical Therapists be Involved in Providing UR?

Expertise

The most important reason can be answered with a question. Who has better clinical understanding of physical therapy services than physical therapists? To truly evaluate treatment and clinical decision making, "like must review like."[2] It only makes sense that reviewers who are experts on the discipline they are reviewing are best qualified to identify fraud and abuse.

Autonomy

For physical therapists to maintain optimal autonomy in the decision-making process for their patients' care, they must make themselves visible on the forefront of UM decision making.

It is vital that we, as physical therapists, engage in review to protect the quality, reimbursement, and reputation of our profession. We need to be leaders in developing our own review criteria, or review organizations outside our profession will do it for us.

Reimbursement denials

UM can be helpful by alerting us as to when reimbursement for our treatment may be jeopardized. If we do not stay abreast of UM regulations, we may find ourselves inadvertently providing patient care on a pro-bono basis, like Anderson Outpatient Center at the beginning of this chapter.

Protecting future resources

As government funds are being stretched to their limit, Medicare must give priority to the most reasonable and necessary cases. This is all the more reason to do your part to help protect against potential fraud and abuse by being involved in screening unnecessary care. As physical therapists become more visible in the health care scene, it is important to protect our reputation, as well as our future.[13]

Hospital cutbacks/manpower shortages

Physical therapists who are unable to prove to reviewers that their patients require their skilled services may find their patients' care inappropriately delegated to less qualified personnel. This realistic snowball effect is already in progress as facilities are hiring fewer physical therapy staff and more ancillary personnel.

No physical therapist is an island

By the nature of your profession, you already are involved with UM every time you document treatment, request reimbursement, or verbally defend your skilled services for treatment.

HOW TO GET TO UM BEFORE IT GETS TO YOU

To conduct optimal and appropriate utilization, it is helpful to adhere to the following strategies:

Understand UR and UM Criteria

Know what your reviewers are looking for. Criteria are commonly documented in the reviewer's policy manual, something that will be helpful for you

TABLE 12.2

COMMON CRITERIA FOR REASONABLE AND NECESSARY SERVICES

1. Is service a documented, accepted treatment based on condition?
2. Does the service require the judgment, knowledge, and skill of the physical therapist, or could ancillary personnel do it?
3. Is there demonstration that a functional or measurable gain has occurred? Are the therapist's skills required to develop a maintenance program?
4. Is there a strong indication that the patient's condition supports the frequency, intensity, and duration of treatment?

Adapted from Abeln SH, Stewart DL. Documenting Outcomes in Physical Therapy. *St. Louis, Mo: Mosby-Year Book Inc; 1993.*

to keep on hand. Table 12.2 presents common questions that reviewers want answered about your services.

The following are criteria for Medicare patients receiving physical therapy services:

- Services relate directly and specifically to an active written treatment program established by the physician or physical therapist providing the services.
- Services are reasonable and necessary to the treatment of an individual illness or injury.[11]

These criteria will be specific to the setting you work in and to your reviewers' expectations. For instance, an example of criteria specific to an inpatient rehabilitation setting can be found in Table 12.3.

These criteria may change depending on which setting is being reviewed. However, a trend is developing as Medicare criteria are beginning to represent the "gold standard" as more health maintenance organizations are being required to adopt these criteria.

As each patient's need varies, so does the interpretation of the criteria that apply. In this case, a physical therapist needs to be skilled at justifying his or her reasons for treatment.

Understanding criteria will also require you to know the background of your reviewers and document according to their level of understanding. In a nutshell, always be able to communicate the answer to the question:

"What does this patient need from physical therapy that no one else can perform that would require my service for $xxx per treatment/day?"

TABLE 12.3

ACUTE INPATIENT REHABILITATION CRITERIA
UTILIZATION REVIEW FORM

Mission review (1 through 3 must be present)

☐ 1. Must have significant physical impairment of recent onset.
☐ 2. Must need close supervision by a physician trained in rehabilitation, availability of 24-hour rehabilitation nursing, and at least two services of a multidisciplinary team.
☐ 3. Must be able to tolerate at least 3 hours of physical therapy, occupational therapy, and/or speech therapy daily.

Continued stay review (must be completed every 7 days)

☐ 1. Patient must show continued improvement toward meeting established goals, and improvement must be noted in a weekly/biweekly team conference report; or
☐ 2. Patient's record must document an unexpected, complicating medical condition that justifies temporary suspension of rehabilitation treatment for no more than 7 days; and
☐ 3. Services cannot be delivered effectively at a lesser level of care.

Adapted from San Joaquin Valley Rehabilitation Hospital, Fresno, Calif, 1996.

Familiarize Yourself with Proper Documentation

This strategy is the most important of all. Documentation is often the only way reviewers can determine if your care is appropriate. In the likely event your reviewer is someone who is not trained in your field, document in layman's terms. Although proper documentation has been presented more thoroughly in Chapter 11, it is important to follow these basic concepts:[8]

- Clearly state the patient's functional limitations, rather than impairments only. Example: Patient is unable to sit at computer for 8 hours due to numbness in LEs induced by static postures.
- Clearly state critical problems, which, when improved, will increase function. Example: Patient is unable to climb stairs without an assistive device due to 3+/5 weakness in hip extension.
- Clearly state measurable goals that focus on treatment intervention that will impact function, not simply signs and symptoms. Example: Patient will ambulate on level surfaces without an assistive device for 100 feet.
- Clearly demonstrate that the patient needs your equipment, supervision, or expertise. For instance, if a patient's condition is not improving, there must be daily documentation proving that an attempt is being made to make progress.[12]

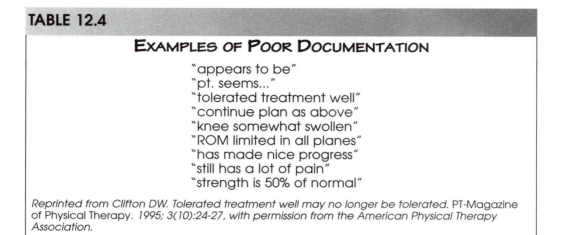

TABLE 12.4

EXAMPLES OF POOR DOCUMENTATION

"appears to be"
"pt. seems..."
"tolerated treatment well"
"continue plan as above"
"knee somewhat swollen"
"ROM limited in all planes"
"has made nice progress"
"still has a lot of pain"
"strength is 50% of normal"

Reprinted from Clifton DW. Tolerated treatment well may no longer be tolerated. PT-Magazine of Physical Therapy. *1995; 3(10):24-27, with permission from the American Physical Therapy Association.*

Example 1: Patient experienced inflammation from weekend activities. Therefore, therapeutic exercise repetitions were decreased by 5.

Example 2: Patient's range of motion has not responded to hip flexor stretches in prone; hip flexor stretch will be modified to standing position.

Don't Let History Repeat Itself—Learn From Others' Mistakes

Pay attention to what the most common reasons for denials are in your department/facility and avoid them. This information may be obtained by talking to your department supervisor, billing personnel, or the reviewers themselves. The following list provides common denials that are prevalent:

- Misuse of procedures or service codes, or "codes that indicate the medical diagnosis of a patient that classifies him or her according to an expected course of care and resultant change in function."[1] For example, patients may be classified under a diagnosis of "fibromyalgia" as opposed to "cervical strain" in order to extend their number of visits. The former treatment diagnosis/code classification allows for more treatments and visits.

- Use of inappropriate goals or treatment methods. Providing lengthy treatment for a patient to change a long-standing functionally dependent status will not benefit either the patient or facility.

- Lengthy stays. A patient who is kept in-house for treatment of a cerebrovascular accident and demonstrates no improvement for several weeks after reaching his or her goals for supervised ambulation provides an example of an excessive length of stay.

- Lack of change in treatment with little or no results. An example of this is the use of "palliative therapies," such as massage, repeatedly for a diagnosis of degenerative joint disease. In this case, the treatment does not address the root of the problem, but only temporarily relieves the symptoms.

- Lack of appropriate cost alternatives. If a patient is safe and independent in performing a therapeutic exercise program, there is no need for the therapist to conduct therapeutic exercise during treatment and charge for therapeutic exercise instruction.

Hospitals may be heavily audited if reviewers notice a pattern of any combination of these criteria being violated.

Communicate with Members of Your Care Team

If your patient is being seen by more than one member of the physical therapy staff, consult with them on your patient's progress. Verify that your treatments and goals coincide with those of your colleagues. This will prevent repetitive, ineffective treatments and will keep you abreast of the patient's changes in function so that no one violates review criteria. This may also involve identifying and resolving problems through a quality improvement system.

PIECING THE PUZZLE TOGETHER

Understanding the niches that all the reviewer roles fit into can be confusing. Many review systems are designed similar to the physical therapy claim triad in Figure 12.1.

The document review paper trail may follow the steps outlined below:
1. Once a physical therapy treatment case (claim for reimbursement) leaves the clinic to be reviewed, it first goes through UR to be assessed for efficacy and effectiveness.
2. If reimbursement is denied at this point, it will be sent back to the physical therapy setting.
3. If UR decides the claim adheres appropriately to criteria, it is sent to claims review.
4. If the claim is rejected at this point, the provider may appeal.

MAKING YOUR CLAIM "APPEALING"

In the event that your claim is rejected, it is important that you, as a provider, assume responsibility to determine what went wrong. The following suggestions offer strategies to protecting reimbursement, quality, and reputation of our treatment decisions:[14]
- Request an explanation for denials.
- Request peer review (practitioner of similar education, licensure, or experiential background).

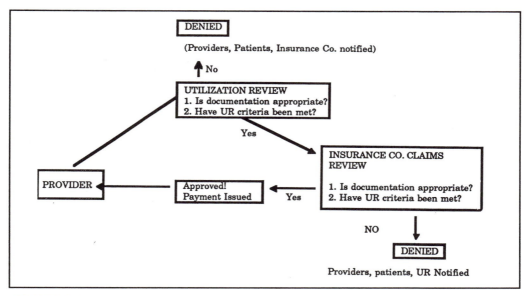

FIGURE 12.1 *Physical therapy claim triad.*

- Always, if all else fails, request an appeal.
- Follow through! It is your responsibility to ensure that clinical decisions are made by the provider and not the reviewer.

As the provider, the burden of proof rests in your hands. We need to demonstrate, through written and verbal communication, evidence of skill and logic of our decision-making process.[11] In the case scenario at the beginning of the chapter, perhaps the therapist would have been reimbursed had he communicated that the wound depth and width were decreasing each month.

EXERCISE YOUR LEADERSHIP IN UM

Now that you've learned about UM, it is up to you to take it a step further. Physical therapists cannot always rely on their supervisors, billing personnel, or utilization reviewers to keep abreast of policies and stipulations required for quality care and reimbursement. Our profession will only suffer if we do not become leaders and get involved in appeals, peer review, review organizations, or at the very least UR/UM current trend information review.[15]

REFERENCES

1. Foto M, Swanson G. Utilization review and managed care. *Rehab Management.* 1993;6(5):123-125.
2. Clifton DW. UR and you. *PT-Magazine of Physical Therapy.* 1995;3(4):38-40.
3. Clifton DW. Who's watching URO's? Part I. *PT-Magazine of Physical Therapy.* 1996;4(11):25-27.
4. Bodenheimer T, Grumbach K. *Understanding Health Policy: A Clinical Approach.* Stamford, Conn: Appleton and Lange; 1995
5. Clifton DW. Utilization management. Whose job is it? *Rehab Management.* 1996;9(5):38-44.
6. Clifton DW. A shift toward utilization management. *PT-Magazine of Physical Therapy.* 1995;3(6):32-35.
7. Boyles-Haubersin, Dawan. Director of Clinical Services, San Joaquin Valley Rehabilitation Hospital, Fresno, Calif. Seminar in Health Care Issues II, lecture notes. March 5, 1996.
8. Abeln S. Improving functional reporting. *PT-Magazine of Physical Therapy.* 1996;4(3):26-30.
9. Clifton DW. Who's watching URO's? Part II. *PT-Magazine of Physical Therapy.* 1996;4(12):26-28.
10. Sinnot M. Critical pathways to success. *PT-Magazine of Physical Therapy.* 1994;2(12):55-63.
11. Clifton DW. Review criteria: cookbook medicine or professional tool? *PT-Magazine of Physical Therapy.* 1995;3(9):37-40.
12. Mondry, Joe. Utilization Reviewer for CCN Medview and physical therapist. Phone interview. January 11, 1997.
13. Clifton DW. PT on the radar screen. *PT-Magazine of Physical Therapy.* 1995;3(2):32-34.
14. Clifton DW. Legal issues in peer review and utilization review. Part 2. *PT-Magazine of Physical Therapy.* 1996;4(2):23-25.
15. Clifton DW. You be the reviewer! *PT-Magazine of Physical Therapy.* 1996;4(6):34-37.
16. Stewart DL, Abeln SH. *Documenting Functional Outcomes in Physical Therapy.* St. Louis, Mo: Mosby-Year Book, Inc; 1993.

TEST YOUR SKILLS

Communication within the physical therapy claim triad at Sports and Orthopedic Rehabilitation, Inc (SORI) leaves much to be desired. All three parties—the contracted workers' compensation insurance company, the utilization reviewers hired by the insurance company, as well as the clinic therapists—are frustrated by the reimbursement process. Upon asking each of these three shareholders who is most at risk in this reimbursement scheme, you will get a different answer from each.

The concerns expressed by the physical therapists at SORI clinic revolve around their lack of reimbursement. The utilization reviewers have rejected low back pain treatment claims on the basis that myofascial release (MFR) "is not medically necessary." The therapists are also frustrated by the external utilization reviewers who did not catch the MFR review criteria discrepancies before the patient was discharged and treatments had occurred. The therapists believe there is not enough time in the workday to sort out these "hassles," as they have too many forms to fill out for each patient.

The utilization reviewers feel they are at risk, as they believe the therapists are accusing them of negligence by limiting the number of visits the workers' compensation patients are allowed. These reviewers argue that they are only making these decisions based on criteria derived from previous outcome reports. Furthermore, the reviewers are frustrated that physical therapists are usually behind on submitting utilization forms for their patients on time and are "generally lazy when it comes to filling out paperwork."

The workers' compensation insurance company feels it is a victim of acting "in good faith," that is, trusting the clinic that the treatment it is paying for is cost efficient and absolutely necessary. The company believes some unnecessary treatments are screened out by UR but is dissatisfied with this "loose regulatory system." The insurance company believes that the utilization reviewers need more rigid accountability to accurately keep up with the mounting claims. Additionally, it is disgruntled about receiving duplicate bills from the clinic for cases that have not yet been reviewed.

(continued on Page 224)

In the scenario on Page 223, where are there possible problems in this system? Consider the perspectives of the physical therapy clinic, the utilization reviewers, and the insurance company claims reviewers. Make a list of possible solutions addressing each problem.

Problems from physical therapy clinic's perspective:

Problems from the utilization reviewer's perspective:

Problems from the workers' compensation insurance company's perspective:

Solutions:

CHECK YOUR RESPONSES

Problems from the physical therapy clinic perspective:
1. Physical therapists have limited time in their day to fill out UR forms.
2. Physical therapists are not informed that they will not be reimbursed for treatment until after the patient is discharged.
3. Physical therapists are not getting reimbursed for "necessary and appropriate" treatment; reviewers have a limited understanding of the clinical significance of myofascial release.

The utilization reviewers' perspective:
1. Utilization reviewers believe therapists are requesting too many visits per patient.
2. Physical therapists are not keeping up with paperwork; therefore, it is difficult to inform them of authorization denials in a timely manner.
3. Physical therapists are not backing up their documentation with proof that their treatment is medically necessary.

Workers' compensation insurance company's perspective:
1. UR reviewers often loosely screen the documentation, and the insurance companies are forced to pay for treatment that is possibly not medically necessary.
2. The billing system from the physical therapy office is unorganized.
3. As payers, they have a limited amount of funds and can only reimburse for treatment that is helping the patient to progress and improve functionally.

Possible solutions:
1. Creation of an "all-inclusive" UR/insurance/Medicare form to decrease physical therapists' paperwork.
2. Purchase and develop computer access to UR and claims review information in the physical therapy clinic (physical therapists can keep abreast of the progression and status of their claims).
3. Educate UR nurses and third-party payers/claims review on documented outcomes showing benefits of myofascial release on low back pain and average number of visits needed.
4. Instate an updated billing system in the clinic's computer with access to claims review/third-party payers.
5. Create an accountability supervisory position within the Joint Commission on the Accreditation of Healthcare to regulate UR effectiveness.
6. The physical therapy clinic could organize an inservice on how to prioritize or create time for proper documentation and UR follow-through.
7. Troubleshoot the billing system for inefficiencies and disorganization, and train billing staff to combat inefficiencies.

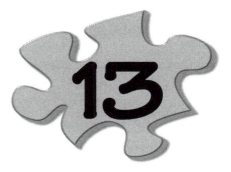

QUALITY MANAGEMENT IN PHYSICAL THERAPY

Noelle Righter-Freer, MPT

A Harvard medical practice study reviewed 30,000 medical records in 51 hospitals in New York State in 1984 and found that in 4% of hospital admissions, the patient experienced a medical injury (a medical problem caused by the management of a disease rather than by the disease itself).

A 1976 US House of Representatives study found that in 1974, unnecessary surgeries led to 11,900 unnecessary deaths (Leape, 1992).

For open heart surgery, 38% of the deaths in smaller-volume hospitals could have been avoided had the procedure been done in larger-volume hospitals (Luft et al, 1990).[1]

These research results are only scratching the surface of poor quality accounts in hospitals today. We don't need to be health care experts to recognize when quality is missing. Most people will agree that the definition of quality is, "I know it when I don't see it." Similarly, we don't need to be health care historians to imagine what health care was like before quality checks were introduced.

Now quality improvement (QI) programs are instated as a branch of utilization review that keeps the patient's best interest in mind. Quality checks have come a long way, as QI for physicians in ancient Mesopotamia meant losing a body part each time they caused their patient harm.[2]

QUALITY—IN THE EYE OF THE BEHOLDER

If we are to implement quality checks, we need to understand what quality is. Like a chameleon, the meaning of quality can take on different shades and is dependent upon which shareholder is viewing it. However, it is important to know each institution's perception, as the quality level of your care depends on who your customer is.[3]

Quality is evaluated from many perspectives at Springfield Rehabilitation Hospital:

If you ask John Daniels, a patient with a cerebrovascular accident, he would say that quality of care is high. "They treated me really nicely at Springfield," he commented on the patient satisfaction survey. "I especially enjoyed my therapist. I could tell that he genuinely cared about what happened to me. He helped me to reach my goal of traveling out-of-state in my motor home with my wife this summer." He completed the survey by marking "excellent" in all areas of performance for the hospital including staff availability, efficiency, timeliness, friendliness, and location convenience.

John's third-party payers may not agree that quality care was provided. "In the future, we will avoid negotiating contracts with Springfield," wrote a claims reviewer in a memo to the hospital. "We have noticed a pattern lacking of cost-effective care, and Mr. Daniels' case is no exception. Funds are not being used efficiently, and patient lengths of stay are too long." The reviewer went on to argue that, although Mr. Daniels was highly satisfied with his treatment, "too much expensive equipment" was ordered to accommodate him with functional activities at home.

Mr. Daniels' therapist was also frustrated by his ability to provide quality care at Springfield. "I feel like my hands are tied. My recommendations for treatment are no longer taken seriously by my director or the insurance companies. My director is only concerned about my productivity. Many insurance companies only care that my patients are able to walk 100 feet without paying attention to their risk for falls. I am forced to discharge them to their homes unsafely. For example, I don't feel that Mr. Daniels should be left in his home alone."

Unfortunately, Mr. Daniels later fell in his home and fractured his hip. He suffered from pneumonia during his hospital stay following ORIF hip surgery. Obviously, Mr. Daniels' idea of quality care was not consistent with his therapist or third-party payers.

QUALITY DEFINED

- **For providers:** "when the freedom is provided to practice the current state of the profession, have autonomy, and provide the patient with optimal care."[2] A provider may view quality therapy as being able to provide gait training, which contributes to the patient's ability to ambulate at home or in the community.
- **For consumers:** "when providers recognize the consumers' perceived needs, are courteous, and communicate concern" and "when the consumers' health status improves with care provided and can function and return to vocation and avocation."[2] A patient may label his or her therapy "quality" when his or her therapist displays sincerity and determination in helping him or her return to playing a game of catch with grandchildren.
- **For third-party payers:** "when there is efficient, effective use of funds, client satisfaction, client return to work/functional level."[2] A payer may recognize quality in therapy when the patient scores therapy high on a patient satisfaction survey, using the most inexpensive resources within the lowest possible number of visits. This may mean educating the patient about a home exercise program rather than giving him or her electrical muscle stimulation to stimulate muscle activity.
- **For field experts:** The Institute of Medicine (in a report to Congress, May 1990): "the degree to which health services for individuals and populations increase the likelihood of the desired outcome and are consistent with the current professional knowledge."[2]

QUALITY IMPROVEMENT STRATEGIES FOR PHYSICAL THERAPISTS

As no setting is perfect, we can always benefit from improving efficiency and efficacy of our physical therapy departments' quality plan. Below is a list of areas in which many departments fall short. Improvement in these areas can lead to greater patient and therapist satisfaction, improved outcomes, increased cost efficiency, and all-around improvement in quality in patient care.[4-9]

- **Make the patient and family a partner.** Involve them in the goal-setting process, and make them responsible to work toward these goals as much as they possibly can on their own.[4]

  It is important to be thorough with the patient and family education process and follow through on their understanding by watching them demonstrate their knowledge.[5] Different ways to enhance this may mean providing information packets about a diagnosis and the rehabilitation process, providing more of an opportunity for face-to-face discussions, and encouraging them to provide written feedback on their care received.[6]

- **Treat the "whole" patient.** When treating a patient for cervical strain, don't ignore his or her need for education about nutrition, regular exercise, or psychological support. This can be accomplished in a timely manner by referring the patient to the proper qualified references while he or she is being seen by you. A quick reminder may be enough to prompt the patient to pursue these needs outside your department.[7,8]
- **Hold yourself accountable to those areas where your facility is falling short of quality.** Use critical pathways as a "report card." This is not intended to promote cookbook therapy, but to compare your patient outcomes to an established measuring stick.[9]
- **Enhance employee contribution.** Ask your staff for input and ideas about what areas need improvement and how to go about addressing them. They may have better insight and fresh creativity to solving problems. This will enhance the team approach to tackling quality issues.

As Tad McKeon suggests, this involves "...investing in employees, taking their suggestions seriously, acting on and implementing employee suggestions, and providing the tools to assist the process."[4]

OPERATIONAL DEFINITIONS

An Endless Array of Acronyms

Although the definition of quality can be ambiguous, the following definitions offer a framework upon which to understand quality existence.

Quality assurance

"A process of comparing actual practice to an existing set of standards and identifying deviations from the norm. It is also used as a mechanism for establishing new standards and criteria, and for defining the optimal, achievable level of competence and quality."[10]

The Joint Commission on Accreditation on Health Care Organizations (JCAHO) defines *quality assurance* (QA) as a "process designed to objectively and systematically monitor and evaluate the quality and appropriateness of patient care, pursue opportunities to improve patient care, and resolve identified problems."[2] Table 13.1 is a sample of a QA annual plan.

QA is now considered outdated, as a new mindset has taken its place: "Quality cannot be assured, only improved."[2] A newer term, implemented in the 1990s, is quality improvement.

TABLE 13.1

QUALITY ASSURANCE ANNUAL PLAN

Criteria	Monitors (tools)	Responsible party(ies)	Date
Patient safety	Check of electrical equipment	Maintenance department	Annually
Patient outcome	Standards by diagnosis	Clinical supervisors	Quarterly
Patient satisfaction	Patient questionnaire	Quality assurance coordinator	Ongoing with monthly summary
Staff performance	Observation of staff in field (home care)	Clinical supervisor	Every 4 months
Utilization of Services	Home Health Agency Record Review committee	External utilization	Quarterly
Department/ program structure	Department policies	Dept. head from another dept. or hospital/agency	Annually

Quality improvement

This term focuses on improving quality outcomes rather than improving the processes designed to improve outcomes. QI has been distinguished from QA as, "[QA] assures society of minimum competence, [QI] offers promises of higher levels of effectiveness, better outcomes, and excellence."[2]

QA involves assembling a team of employees from different departments to instate a QI program, rather than requiring employees to follow a program that is sent down from the top. The employees identify the outcomes they believe to measure quality and then proceed to create a QI checklist necessary to achieve these outcomes. This approach is believed to be more effective than when supervisors simply delegate quality tasks to their staff.[4]

Outcomes

Outcomes are defined as the "status of the patient after care has been provided; end result of care." Outcomes, otherwise known as QI "goals," should be written as time-specific, measurable, and in functional terms.[2] See Chapter

---

TABLE 13.2

CHECKLIST FOR PATIENTS RECEIVING WORKERS' COMPENSATION

Check each of the following:

_____Initial limited functional capacity
_____Write to physician
_____Contact the adjuster
_____Contact the employer
_____Job description
_____Attempt to treat five times per week
_____Case closed summary
_____Returned to work
_____Did not return to work
_____Contacted
_____Discharge
_____Total patient cost
_____Number of treatments
_____Length of treatments

Reprinted from Hunter SJ, Olsen B, Stewart L. TQM in PT. PT-Magazine of Physical Therapy. 1993; 1(7):54-85, with permission from the American Physical Therapy Association.

---

10 for a thorough presentation of outcomes management. Table 13.2 presents several outcomes in the variables "return to work," "total patient cost," and "number of treatments."

Quality management

Quality management (QM) is "a continuous function to systematically assess and improve health care as a whole or any of its specific clinical, administrative, or support functions."[2] This is a management system that measures, monitors, and strives to improve quality outcomes of the traditional and emerging system. QM offers a team approach through collaboration of health care disciplines to formulate a problem list and solutions for improving quality in the department. Quality management is the system that manages the process of quality improvement, continuous quality improvement (CQI), and total quality management (TQM).

Continuous quality improvement/total quality management

These terms connote "systems that promote continual scrutiny of a product or service to make it better primarily through teamwork and supportive management."[11] They involve deductive reasoning, specific outcomes, and outcome improvement. TQM is a term that evolved from CQI. As another form of QI, the two terms are often used interchangeably.

The intention of all the above processes of QA, QI, CQI, and TQM are to identify and "fix" quality shortcomings in the health care setting. The processes of QI, TQM, and CQM are all demonstrated in a sample of a therapist's checklist (see Table 13.2). This checklist is included in each patient chart to remind therapists of tasks to complete in improving patient outcomes.

Confusion can set in with differing perspectives and regulations of quality. A poorly instated quality improvement process will do nothing to improve problems in your busy systems, it will only create them. Consequently, it is helpful to streamline goals and approaches according to the four critical elements for quality care when implementing QI. These can serve as a solid model for any practice and should keep in mind the employer, the payer, the patient, and the provider.[2]

STEPS TO QUALITY IMPROVEMENT

No matter who the reviewers are, most will agree on the following components for improving an organization's quality. They are outlined by Forer[12] as

1. Identification of potential problems (indicators)
2. Objective assessment of possible causes
3. Implementation of decisions or actions designed to eliminate identified problems (strategies)
4. Monitoring activities to ensure desired results have been obtained
5. Documentation to substantiate that quality has led to improved patient care

To carry out this plan of quality, you must be aware of indicators and strategies. These are operational definitions important to executing a plan of quality care.

Indicators

Indicators are "measurements of criteria selected to evaluate the quality of care."[13] These criteria change and are specific to the type of patient care given. They are most commonly manifest in terms of "outcomes" (ie, lengths of stay, re-admissions, costs per patient discharge).

One example of how indicators are most currently being followed is through the Health Plan Employer Data and Information Set. This is a software program in which indicators are collected in the form of outcomes data and measured. The National Committee for Quality Assurance, a committee

TABLE 13.3	
EXAMPLES OF INDICATORS AND STRATEGIES FOR AN OUTPATIENT SETTING	
Indicators	**Strategies**
Patient complaints	Identify root of problem; create steps to avoid a future mistake
Lack of subjective/ objective documentation changes	Change treatment approach; consult or refer
Lack of short-term/ long-term goal achievement	Make goals feasible; change treatment approach
Lack of evidence of patient/ family communication and education	Instate patient education program; require the patient/family to recall or demonstrate knowledge

that accredits health maintenance organizations, is taking the lead in implementing this new program. Eventually, these reviewed indicators will be important to managed care organizations, corporate purchasers, state regulatory agencies, consumers, purchasers of HMO plans, as well as health providers themselves.[14]

If these measurements of criteria drop below the threshold of what is decided as an acceptable level of quality, then correction needs to be implemented. Correction is then carried out through a strategy.

Strategy

A *strategy* is the process of devising and implementing a plan to reach a goal. Strategies provide a "plan of attack" to bring the indicators back up to an acceptable standard (Table 13.3).

Regulation of "Acceptable Levels of Quality"

Staying on top of indicator recognition and strategy implementation is easier said than done. It is one challenge to arrive at a consensus on what quality is, but it is an even greater challenge to remain accountable to it.[2] Some facilities have their own system of internal review, often in the form of peer review or "mock reviews" before external reviewers evaluate them for continued accreditation.

However, the law of human nature causes us to prioritize situations that lay closest to our personal interests. Most commonly in QM, these priorities are enforced by pressure applied by external, rather than internal, reviews. These external forces take the form of third-party payers (ie, through denied claims), patient satisfaction survey results, referring doctors, accreditation standards, and even litigation threats. Feedback from these sources provides a checks and balances system between all interested parties involved in quality care.[15]

More formal organizations that require regular structured accountability through audits and evaluations include the following:[2]

- Federal governmental agencies (Health Care Financing Administration, Medicare)
- State governmental agencies (Medicaid, MediCal)
- Professional associations (APTA)
- Independent accrediting agencies (JCAHO, Commission of Accreditation of Rehabilitation Facilities)

These organizations generally require documented proof that health care facilities are providing quality care. If hospitals want to keep their accreditation, they are required to undergo quality checks, generally once every 2 years, and even more frequently if an area of quality is questionable within the facility. This will generally involve a site visit from two employees representing the accrediting organization who, through observation and documentation review, fill out a "report card" stating whether or not the facility measures up to specific criteria.

An example of such criteria is outlined in Table 13.4 in the 1996 JCAHO *Standards for Rehabilitation Care and Services*. Evidence of performance to measure these criteria are measured by the following examples:

1. Interviews with rehabilitation services staff
2. Policies and procedures addressing rehabilitation care planning
3. Medical records[16]

The following is a true account of a case, Wilson vs. Blue Cross of Southern California, which entered the justice system in 1990:[17]

A 17-year-old patient was referred by her physician to a psychiatric hospital with a diagnosis of depression, drug dependency, and anorexia. Her attending physician decided her condition was appropriate for 3 or 4 weeks of inpatient care. Her insurance company decided that she should be discharged after 10 days, that any further treatment would be determined unreasonable and medically unnecessary. Soon after she was discharged from the hospital, she committed suicide. Her family filed suit against the insurer, the review organization, and the physician. Lower courts found the treating physician responsible for the premature discharge. However, the court of appeals found the third-party payers liable for improper peer review.

TABLE 13.4

1996 JCAHO STANDARDS FOR REHABILITATION CARE AND SERVICES

Standard TX.6: Qualified professionals provide rehabilitation services consistent with professional licensure laws, regulation, registration, and certification.

Standard TX.6.1: A rehabilitation plan, developed by qualified professionals and based on assessment of patient needs, guides provision of rehabilitation services.

Standard TX.6.2: Qualified professionals implement the rehabilitation plan with the patient and his or her family, social network, or support system.

Standard TX.6.3: Rehabilitation restores, improves, or maintains the patient's optimal level of functioning, self-care, self-responsibility, independence, and quality of life.

Standard TX.6.4: The patient's readiness to end rehabilitation services is determined based on written discharge criteria.

We can all learn from the many mistakes that have occurred in issuing quality care. We must keep abreast of external regulations affecting our care and, most of all, keep the patient's best interest in mind. Know to whom you are accountable in your facility and what his or her requirements are. If you see quality lacking, report it and offer your suggestions to solve it. This may require us to assume an assertive role in patient advocacy. After all, your patient is your most important consumer!

REFERENCES

1. Bodenheimer TS, Grumbach K. *Understanding Health Policy: A Clinical Approach.* Stamford, Conn: Appleton & Lange; 1995.
2. Stewart D, Abeln S. *Documenting Functional Outcomes in Physical Therapy.* St. Louis, Mo: Mosby; 1993.
3. McIntosh G, Mayo MC, Stymiest PJ. Implementing CQI: Measuring levels of service quality at physiotherapy clinics. *Physiotherapy Canada.* 1994;46(3):178-189.
4. McKeon T. Total quality management is everyone's responsibility: A process management approach. *Home Health Care Management and Practice.* 1996;8(5):68-72.
5. Ryan NP, Wade JC, Nice A, Shenefelt H, Shepard K. Physical therapists' perceptions of family involvement in the rehabilitation process. *Physiotherapy Research International.* 1996;1(3):159-179.

6. Toczek-McPeake A, Matthews M. Quality management: A survey of client and career satisfaction with speech pathology and physiotherapy services in a rehabilitation setting. *Journal of Cognitive Rehabilitation.* 1995;13(5):12-18.

7. Berger D. Process-oriented vs. holistic-style physical therapy. *Clinical Management in Physical Therapy.* 1989;9(1):9-11.

8. Broy SB. A 'whole patient' approach to managing osteoporosis. *Journal of Musculoskeletal Medicine.* 1996;13(2):15-30.

9. Stahl DA. Critical pathways in subacute care. *Nursing Management.* 1995;26(9):16-18.

10. Chauhaun L, Hutching D, LePoerk K, Murphy P. Quality assurance manual. *Clinical Management.* 1986;6(5):28-31.

11. Hunter S, Olsen B, Stewart L. TQM in PT. *PT-Magazine of Physical Therapy.* 1993;1(7):54-85.

12. Forer S. Changing management structures. *Rehab Management.* 1994;8(4):33-37.

13. D'Aquila N, Habegger D, Willwerth E. Converting a QA Program to CQI. *Nursing Management.* 1994; 25(10):68-71.

14. Grimaldi PL. Monitoring managed care's quality. *Nursing Management.* 1995;26(9):12-15.

15. Jackson-Frankl KA. The language and meaning of quality. *Nursing Administration Quarterly.* 1990;14(3):52-65.

16. JCAHO. *Standards for Rehabilitation Care and Services, 1996.* Oakbrook Terrace, Ill: Joint Commission on Accreditation of Health Care Organizations; 1996.

17. Clifton D. Legal issues in peer review and utilization review. Part 2. *PT-Magazine of Physical Therapy.* 1996;4(2):23-25.

TEST YOUR SKILLS

Exercise your Eye for Quality Care

Presented below is a table listing indicators to identify areas for possible improvement in an orthopedic outpatient setting. Next to these indicators are corresponding solutions to address quality deficits in these areas. Fill in the empty boxes with the appropriate indicators or their corresponding strategies (see Table 13.3 for examples).

Problems	Indicators	Strategies
1. Numerous referral source complaints, re: patient care	1. Number of referral source complaints	1.
2. Lack of staff participation in ongoing education	2.	2. Encourage staff inservice and continuing education hours
3. Lack of patient continuity of care with staff members	3. Number of therapists, PTAs, and aides assigned per patient throughout the continuum of care at the facility	3.
4. Loss of insurance contracts due to noncompetitive fees	4. Billing charges' consistency with community standards	4.
5. High number of authorization denials	5.	5. Appeal to claims reviewer for reimbursing certification denial
6. High patient noncompliance	6. Patient compliance rate	6.
7. Hospital annual budget exceeded	7.	7. Identify key waste areas for budget and make appropriate cuts
8. High rate of extended lengths of stay	8.	8. Re-evaluate treatment approach
9. High rate of physical therapist overtime	9. Time spent per physical therapist on ancillary tasks	9.
10. High patient disability reoccurrence rate	10.	10. Ensure patient's independence and compliance with home program

CHECK YOUR RESPONSES

Some possible responses might include:

1. Strategy: Identify areas of communication breakdown with physicians; develop rapport.
2. Indicator: Number of inservice and continuing education hours used.
3. Strategy: Assign one physical therapist and one support staff member per patient.
4. Strategy: Research competitive prices and instate competitive and appropriate prices.
5. Indicator: Number of claims denied.
6. Strategy: Be assertive and firm to discourage missed appointments; identify communication deficits between patient and staff.
7. Indicator: Total facility expenditures on equipment and inventory per month.
8. Indicator: Number of lengths of stay exceeding variance.
9. Strategy: Delegate tasks to support staff.
10. Indicator: Number of patients returning to treatment after discharge.

THE ROLE OF PHYSICAL THERAPY IN PREVENTION AND WELLNESS

Judith M. Reposo, MPT

Dana Stypula, MPT

Sarah is a 60-year-old nurse suffering from severe and debilitating back pain. She has a history of degenerative disk disease, as well as numerous falls over the past 30 years. She is in constant pain and has been unable to work for the past 6 years. Accompanied by her husband, she has come to see Matthew, a physical therapist at the Oak Grove Physical Therapy Clinic, for an evaluation. Matthew sees that Sarah walks poorly, requiring the assistance of both her husband and a cane. During the course of the evaluation, Matthew discovers that Sarah's calf muscles are very tight, limiting her ability to dorsiflex her ankles. He thinks that this is one factor contributing to her frequent falls. When he attempts to instruct Sarah's husband in techniques he can use to help Sarah stretch her legs, her husband states he will not have the time to help her stretch because he works two jobs and performs all the chores in their household because Sarah is unable to do them. Sarah's insurer is requiring this evaluation before it will authorize payment for the spinal stimulator her physician wishes to implant to control her pain, as medication is no longer effective. Matthew is frustrated by what he sees as a poor prognosis for Sarah's future physical abilities.

M atthew is faced with attempting to treat a patient without much hope for improvement in her condition. But what if Sarah had received physical therapy after her first fall, including instruction on how to improve her strength and flexibility to prevent further injuries? Or what if she had received instruction in fitness strategies and proper patient lifting techniques at the hospital where she worked, prior to her first back pain symptoms and fall? Her suffering, her family's suffering, and the expense of implant surgery and rehabilitation could well have been prevented.

WHAT IS PREVENTION?

The purpose of prevention in health care is to avoid or limit complications and disabilities from disease or injury.

Prevention has three stages:

1. *Primary prevention:* The prevention of injury and disease to those individuals who are still well and healthy.[1-3] Suzy Johnson, a seventh-grade student at Learning a Lot Elementary School, attends her daily physical education class in which she must participate in running, swimming, and group sports.

2. *Secondary prevention:* The screening and early detection of symptoms, which seeks to prevent further damage once an injury or illness has occurred.[1-4] Dan Thomas, who has had paraplegia since an accident 4 years ago, is referred to the physical therapist for his biannual postural screening exam.

3. *Tertiary prevention:* Interventions to limit further disability and early death, and to maximize independence with disability.[1-3] Marty Reyes, a 45-year-old man with a history of chronic rheumatoid arthritis, sees his physical therapist twice a week to prevent associated deformities and to allow him to remain independent in his daily activities.

Prevention and the Medical Model

When physical therapy began as a profession during World War I, therapists worked as *reconstruction aides*, caring for the injured and ill under the guidance of physicians. Physicians serve as the primary entry for patients into health care, referring patients to other health care personnel for certain aspects of their care, including physical therapy. Following this medical model requires intervening after the insult has occurred, at the tertiary prevention stage.[2-3]

Other health professions practice prevention as well, at different levels. Nurses have a long history in wellness and health promotion (ie, diabetes screening and education, breast self-exam education, and providing information about topics ranging from premenstrual syndrome and stress, to osteoporosis).[4] Interestingly, dentistry has long focused on prevention. In fact, one dental third-party payer covers 100% of preventive procedures and only 50% to 80% of tertiary treatments (ie, crowns, fillings).[2-3]

The *medical model* approach to prevention and health promotion attempts to effect change in patients' high-risk lifestyles by working with individual patients.[1] This approach allows for one-on-one education of patients, assisting them in making lifestyle changes that promote good health. The *public health model* seeks to make change on a larger scale. Examples include public information campaigns to reduce tobacco and alcohol consumption and poor dietary habits, HIV prevention education in schools, and banning cigarette smoking in the workplace. As lower income status is associated with increased morbidity and mortality rates, societal measures to improve the standard of living broadly address prevention. To truly effect change, a combined approach is needed.

The Current Role of Physical Therapists in Prevention

The American Physical Therapy Association's (APTA) *Model Definition of Physical Therapy for State Practice Acts* includes prevention and wellness in its definition of physical therapy, stating that the role of the physical therapist includes "preventing injury, impairments, functional limitations, and disability, including the promotion and maintenance of fitness, health, and quality of life in all age groups."[5] The official liability carrier of the APTA now covers wellness services provided by physical therapists.[2,3,6] Physical therapists often serve as educators, making us well-suited to play a key role in prevention and wellness.[7] The APTA House of Delegates "recognizes that physical therapists are uniquely qualified to assume leadership positions in efforts to prevent injury and disability, and fully supports the positive roles that physical therapists... play in the promotion of healthy lifestyles, wellness, and injury prevention."[8] Physical therapists are taking part in prevention and wellness in a variety of ways. We promote wellness through education about lifestyle, exercise, ensuring safety, and workplace evaluations. Often, physical therapists participate in worksite employee evaluations to educate on proper body mechanics, nutrition, and physical fitness.[9]

Prevention and the Aging Population

In 1995, the APTA published a position paper in the *PT Bulletin* entitled, *Physical Therapy and the Aging Population*.[9] Its purpose is to assist in developing recommendations for executive and legislative action to maintain and

improve the well-being of this population. The APTA believes that it is possible to define an affordable package of restorative and preventative physical therapy services that would result in significant health care cost savings. Such a program, as defined by the APTA, includes such preventive measures:
- Osteoporosis and arthritis intervention initiatives
- Programs aimed at decreasing falls in older adults
- Educational services for patients and caregivers on disease processes and the necessary measures to care for their loved ones at home

An example of primary prevention directed at this group was presented at the 1996 Combined Sections Meeting in Atlanta, Ga.[10] A program on osteoporosis was sponsored by Geriatrics, Women's Health, APTA Department of Women's Initiatives, and the National Osteoporosis Foundations. The *Building Better Bones* program's target audience was unique. Not only was it directed at APTA members, but it was also marketed to the public. Forty men and women from the Atlanta area enrolled to find out what they could do to prevent and manage osteoporosis, as well as to learn the role that physical therapy plays in this topic. A panel of multidisciplinary experts spoke on the topic, followed by a participatory exercise session. Many participants felt empowered as they gained both insight and guidance in this area.

Below is an example of secondary prevention targeted at an older patient:

Mrs. Tumble is referred by her physician for treatment of low back injury. During the interview with the patient, it is discovered that she has a history of hypertension (which is managed with diuretics), diabetes, degenerative joint disease in both knees, and bilateral cataracts. In addition, her accompanying daughter reveals that her mother has fallen several times during the past 3 months but, because of her lack of injury, she fails to recall the incidents.

In the case of Mrs. Tumble, there is a risk of serious injury, and a comprehensive strategy of identifying risk factors is an integral part of her treatment.[11] By screening a high-risk individual and pinpointing problem areas associated with falling episodes (Table 14.1), an extensive program aimed at education on household safety tips, such as using night lights and removing throw rugs, can substantially decrease the patient's risk of serious injury.

Prevention and Wellness go to Work

In 1994, approximately 2.5 million workers suffered injuries in the workplace that resulted in at least 1 day away from work beyond the day of the

TABLE 14.1

Fall-related Physical Examination: What to Check For

Postural blood pressure: Orthostatic hypotension
Mental status evaluation: Delirium, dementia, depression
Visual assessment: Visual acuity, cataracts, glaucoma, macular degeneration
Cardiac evaluation: Arrhythmias, valvular disorders, bruits
Neurologic evaluation: Focal deficits, peripheral neuropathy, tremor
Musculoskeletal evaluation: Muscular weakness, arthritis
Podiatric evaluation: Nail disorders, toe deformities, condition of footwear

Adapted from Tideiksaar R. Geriatrics. 1996; 51(2):46.

injury.[12] Of those, 44% were from "bodily reaction and exertion," which includes overexertion, reactions (ie, slips, twisting), and repetitive motion. Repetitive motion injuries (ie, from grasping tools, typing, scanning groceries) resulted in absences with a median of 18 days missed. Between 1983 and 1992, cumulative trauma disorders increased by 1126%, resulting in an increase in the number of workers' compensation claims, increased absenteeism, impaired productivity, and increased employee turnover.[13]

Physical therapists offer unique skills to combat these injuries. Physical therapists serve as workplace injury consultants, giving suggestions for ergonomic improvements while providing education on posture, exercise, and improving positioning while using equipment. With these programs, business and industry seek to reduce on-the-job injuries.[14-15] According to the US Labor Department's Bureau of Labor Statistics, the number of employers using this approach is growing.[16]

Tom Krajecki, district safety manager at Ryder Truck Rental, Inc, located in Harvey, Ill, has seen a substantial decrease in occupational injuries and "sick" days since the implementation of Jean Lane's Mercy Works program.[17] Lane is a physical therapist and industrial service coordinator at Chicago's Mercy Hospital. At Ryder, she measured workers' initial physical condition, provided educational sessions, and prescribed individually based exercise programs. The employees were retested approximately 3 to 4 months later and showed great improvements in physical condition, general health, strength to resist a crippling injury, and body mechanics. The employees saw the program progression as educational and empowering, and they understood the effects of cumulative trauma. In addition to the knowledge gained, evidence exists that supports that workers experienced an increase in abdominal strength and trunk stabilization.

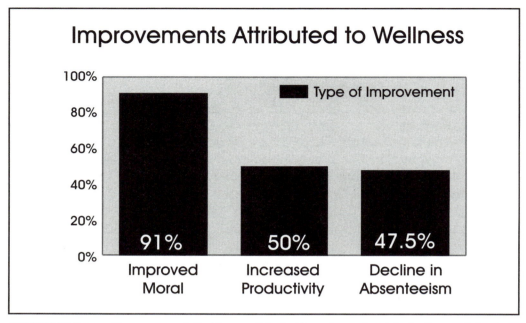

FIGURE 14.1 *Types of improvements that have attributed to wellness. Reprinted with permission from* Wellness Program Management Advisors *newsletter; 1996.*

Wellness programs in the workplace can also bring health promotion education to people who might not otherwise obtain the information. Men make 150 million fewer visits to the doctor per year than women, while suffering premature death, disability, and dying an average of 7 years younger than women.[18] They are more likely to develop conditions associated with lifestyle choices like tobacco use, alcohol consumption, and risk taking. Research shows that most men lack the health care knowledge needed to reduce these mortality and disability rates. Bringing the information to the worksite makes it more accessible to these men.

Wellness programs have been found to have a significant impact on America's workplaces, improving employee morale, job performance, and decreasing absentee rates and health care costs (Figure 14.1).[19] A study sponsored by Wellness Program Management Advisors reported that seven out of 10 wellness professionals surveyed stated that implementing a program at their worksite improved employee morale. In addition, of the respondents who credited wellness programs with specific improvements, half found increased productivity, and 47.5% reported a decline in absenteeism. Beth-Ann Kerber, editor of the *Wellness Program Management Advisors* newsletter, stated, "Wellness programs are being found to have an effect on a company's bottom

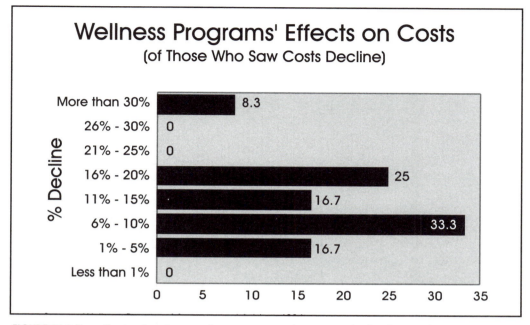

FIGURE 14.2 *The effects of costs on wellness programs that saw a decline in costs in 1996. Reprinted with permission from* Wellness Program Management Advisors *newsletter; 1996.*

line. Approximately 22% of respondents said the wellness program decreased their health care costs—some by 30%" (Figure 14.2).

Backing Prevention with Back School

In the early 1970s, back schools were introduced.[20] While their structure varies from site to site, their basic aim is to change behaviors that induce or create back pain and injury. They use concepts of strength, fitness, proper body mechanics (ie, lifting techniques), and stress management skills. They may be primary or secondary in nature.

Overall, back schools have proved effective. A primary prevention back school for bus drivers in Holland resulted in an average decline in absenteeism of 6 days per year.[20] A physical therapy department, in conjunction with an employee health services department of a hospital, implemented a back care education program for the hospital's employees. In the year following implementation of its program, the costs of back injuries of workers decreased from $272,751 to $72,296.[21] A study of the effects of a secondary prevention program, which included both physical and behavioral therapy for nurses with a history of low back pain, showed that the nurses in the intervention group showed significant improvements over those in the control group in many

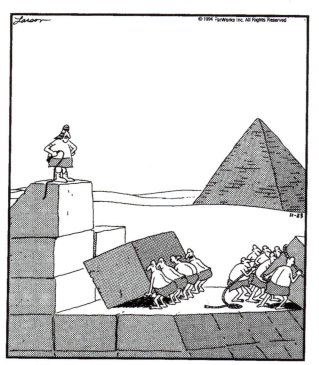

"Remo! Lift with your knees, not your back!"

areas, including pain intensity, sleep quality, anxiety, fatigue, and ability to perform daily activities.[22] Back school in conjunction with a rehabilitation or exercise program has been shown to be more effective than back school alone.[23-24]

EFFECTIVENESS AND COSTS OF PREVENTION AND WELLNESS

In addition to the examples previously mentioned, there is much more documentation of the benefits of preventive interventions.[1] Coronary heart disease mortality rates declined by 32% between 1968 and 1981. This decline had more to do with public health interventions regarding tobacco use and the benefits of a low-fat diet than with advances in cardiac care. Implementation of a back school by a physical therapist at a glass factory reduced the worker injury rate by 70%.[25] Another hospital worksite wellness program resulted in a 67% improvement in the health status of the participants, as defined in Figure 14.1.[26]

Does prevention save money? It is difficult to get a clear answer. Like all services, health promotion and wellness programs cost money. One dollar spent on prenatal care saves $3.38 in newborn intensive care, while $1.00 spent in measles-mumps-rubella immunizations saves $13.40.[1] Some measures save money and some do not. After implementation of an injury prevention program at a Chicago truck rental company, the cost of lost work days declined from $2953 in all of 1995 to $550 for the first 6 months of 1996.[17] Costs of lost worker productivity, absenteeism, and staff turnover are difficult to calculate.[27]

While monetary savings are not always easy to measure, we intuitively understand that prevention is a wise investment.[28] We increase the value of the health care dollar by improving the quality of life of our patients and reducing suffering, not only preventing the need for more expensive medical interventions. Our ethical obligation is not to save money, but to treat our patients to the best of our ability while using resources prudently.

Payment for preventive and wellness services by third-party payers (insurers) is limited.[3,7] Most will pay for immunizations, well baby care, mammograms, and some other routine screening procedures, but not for preventive physical therapy services. Many wellness programs are paid for out-of-pocket by the participants. Additional documentation of the benefits of preventive services provided by physical therapists is needed to increase third-party payer reimbursement. However, third-party payers are not the only alternative. Employers are increasingly recognizing the benefits of paying for wellness and preventive care programs. Promotion of these benefits to employers can increase their willingness to underwrite physical therapy prevention services.

CHARACTERISTICS OF A SUCCESSFUL PREVENTION PROGRAM

Get Into the Groove

Lack of motivation is the primary cause of noncompliance for many patients. By using a humanistic model that focuses more on individual goals, as opposed to all-encompassing program goals, participation is more long-lasting.[29] In addition, by approaching the program with gusto, the leader's enthusiasm will catch on.

Expand Your Horizons

By integrating several related elements into the program, such as nutrition, psychological support, and physical activity, the individual needs of the participant are met in a well-rounded and expansive manner.[30]

Show That You Care

This type of behavior includes characteristics such as flexibility, acceptance, unconditional support, listening, friendship, and competence.[30] These attributes provide the participant with a feeling of true understanding and empathy, instilling trust and resulting in a more productive patient-therapist relationship.

Empower with Power

The term empowerment is defined as "a process of helping people to assert control over the factors that affect their lives."[30] By helping participants to realize that they have power and educating them on how to exercise that power, they feel more in control of their own lives.

NEW POSSIBILITIES AND TRENDS

In addition to providing services in the workplace, physical therapists operate fitness centers and programs associated with physical therapy clinics across the country. Some programs specialize in working with specific populations. Judy Devereaux, a physical therapist in Albuquerque, NM, opened Fifty 'n' Fit, a health club for the fastest growing segment of the population, people 50 years and older, in 1991.[31] She also owns a physical therapy practice that operates in conjunction with the health club. Devereaux has trained her staff of personal trainers, and their services are available to club members. Physical therapy patients use the gym as part of their rehabilitation process; and when they have completed their course of therapy, they can continue to improve their fitness levels as health club members.

In the Detroit suburb of Farmington Hills, Mich, the Total Rehabilitation and Athletic Conditioning Center (TRACC) operates as a satellite physical therapy clinic and department of Botsford General Hospital.[7] In addition to offering one-on-one physical therapy treatment sessions, TRACC offers a variety of health promotion and wellness programs, such as an arthritis water program, prenatal water aerobics class, and kinetics class (an exercise program designed for people with a history of low back problems or arthritis).

Opportunities to work with specific populations in fitness programs abound. Julie Pauls, MS, PT, focuses on women's health at the Women's Atrium in Houston Northwest Medical Center.[31] There, she has taught classes on back care, pelvic floor dysfunction, prepared childbirth, and special back problems of pregnancy. The center includes a fitness center, educational facilities, and obstetrical and neonatal units. Karen Johnstone, PT, coaches the Motor City Wheelers Swim Club, a program for children and young adults with spinal disabilities. The club focuses on the physical fitness and emotional well-being of the athletes as they compete in regular and national meets.

Sean P. Gallagher, PT, is the founder of Performing Arts Physical Therapy.[32] He contracts with dance companies to provide services to the performers. Having a physical therapist's expertise available to dancers helps them prevent injuries, as well as offering timely and appropriate care should injuries occur.

HealthTouch is a system that was designed to extend preventive care to patients via computer.[33] As patients participate actively in their own health care, the usefulness of computers becomes increasingly apparent. Computers provide patients with individualized information to increase motivation, track patient needs, and facilitate communication between the patient and the health care professional. This system was donated by family physicians and placed in 29 randomly selected primary care practices in Virginia for 1 year. The physicians felt that it was successful in that it provided an efficient way to enhance the doctor-patient interaction and provide patient-specific educational materials. The program has been successful, as the authors found that completion of the recommended prevention steps was generally high. This system is well-accepted by patients, can be installed in the busy practice setting with little effort, and is effective in achieving consistency of preventive care.

Prevention information for physical therapists and patients alike can be provided via the Internet.[34-35] *PT Bulletin* reported the story of two families with disabled children with similar medical issues who met on a website devoted to helping parents such as themselves. One family lived in Texas and the other in Canada. Through their correspondence, they met a physical therapist who arranged for them to attend a workshop together on functional motor skills education and training for their children.

INCORPORATING PREVENTION AND WELLNESS INTO YOUR PRACTICE

Offer Your Vast Knowledge

You worked so hard to complete the requirements of your physical therapy education and now you finally wonder what to do with all that you learned. Give some to your patients! Help them to help themselves.

What's Going on Around You?

Identify the risk factors that predominate in your patient population. Consult the literature, conduct your own research, and ask your co-workers what they are doing to prevent these issues in their patients.

Facilitate Worksite Wellness in Your Own Area

Investigate the primary injuries and health risks of your fellow staff members and initiate a wellness program addressing those specific areas. Make it fun and enjoyable for everyone.

Clean Up Your Own Backyard

By keeping yourself fit and preventing illness and injury in your own life, you can be a role model for your patients. Your ability to speak from personal experience will help keep them motivated.

SUMMARY

Today, physical therapists are taking on many roles in prevention, from patient education to worksite wellness evaluation and programs. *Primary prevention* (preventing injury and disease in those who are healthy), *secondary prevention* (screening and early detection), and *tertiary prevention* (the intervention to limit further complication of disability) are the three types of prevention in which physical therapists can play a role. Physical therapists have long functioned in the tertiary realm, but are well suited to working in the primary and secondary levels by our knowledge of pathophysiology, biomechanics, and exercise, as well as our background as patient educators. Prevention benefits the patient and the payer, while making good use of the physical therapist's expertise. Reimbursement for these services can be out-of-pocket, via insurer, or from an employer for a worksite program. If you are not currently implementing prevention programs in your workplace, the ideas in this chapter may provide a place to start.

REFERENCES

1. Bodenheimer T, Grumbach K. *Understanding Health Policy: A Clinical Approach.* Stamford, Conn: Appleton and Lange; 1995.
2. Anderson S. *Preventive care: are physical therapists missing the boat? Do we need to shift the paradigm again?* American Physical Therapy Association Combined Sections Meeting. February 14, 1997.
3. McLaughlin C. A step in the "well" direction: PTs take aim for prevention and wellness. *ADVANCE for Physical Therapists.* 1997;8(12):10-11.
4. Johny A, Bille DA. On the scene: section III—wellness promotion. *Nursing Administration Quarterly.* 1987;11(3):61-65.
5. *Model Definition of Physical Therapy for State Practice Acts.* BOD-03-95-24-64. Fairfax, Va: American Physical Therapy Association; 1995.
6. Sterneck J. Liability awareness: Beyond the borders of hands-on care. *PT-Magazine of Physical Therapy.* 1997;5(3):28-31.
7. Woods EN. Making TRACCs: toward a healthier community. Total Rehabilitation and Athletic Conditioning Center. *PT-Magazine of Physical Therapy.* 1995;3(6):40-44, 46, 48-52.
8. *Physical therapists in health promotion and wellness.* House of Delegates HOD 06-93-25-50. Fairfax, Va: American Physical Therapy Association; 1993.
9. Ketter P. Health status, health services utilization will be major issues of PTs at WHCoA. *PT Bulletin.* 1995;10(16):6-7.
10. Woods EN. Building better bones: managing and preventing osteoporosis. *PT-Magazine of Physical Therapy.* 1996;4(5):41-42.
11. Tideiksaar R. Preventing falls: how to identify risk factors, reduce complications. *Geriatrics.* 1996; 51(2):43-46,49-50,53-55.
12. Characteristics of injuries and illnesses resulting in absences from work, 1994. Press release issued May 8, 1996. Bureau of Labor Statistics, U.S. Department of Labor. http://stats.bls.gov/pub/news.release/osh2.tx. April 12, 1997.
13. Dal Pra V. Two Illinois hospitals form task force for repetitive motion injuries. *PT Bulletin.* 1995;10(16):10-11.
14. Clauser G. Hands-on prevention: advising the chronic keyboarder. *Physical Therapy Today.* 1995;8-9, 11-13.
15. Huhn R, Volski R. Primary prevention programs for business and industry. *Phys Ther.* 1985;65:1840-1844.
16. Government sees growing demand for physical therapy through 2005. *PT Bulletin.* 1997;12(8):1.
17. Aron LJ. Outcomes measurement in injury prevention programs. *Rehab Management.* 1996;9(4):74, 76-77.
18. Men lack health care knowledge. *PT Bulletin.* 1995; 10(25):26.
19. Kerber BA. Study confirms the benefits of workplace wellness programs. *PT Bulletin.* 1996;11(19):7.
20. Nordin M, Cedraschi C, Falague F, Roux EB. Back schools in the prevention of chronicity. *Bailliere's Clinical Rheumatology.* 1992;6:685-703.

21. Ryden LA, Molgaard CA, Bobbitt S. Benefits of a back care and light duty health promotion program in a hospital setting. *J Community Health.* 1988; 13(4):222-230.

22. Linton S, Bradley LA, Jensen I, Spangfolt, E, Sundell L. The secondary prevention of low back pain: a controlled study with follow-up. *Pain.* 1989;36(2):197-207.

23. Donchin M, Woolf O, Kaplan L, Floman Y. Secondary prevention of low-back pain: a clinical trial. *Spine.* 1990;15(12):1317-1320.

24. DiFabio RP. Efficacy of comprehensive rehabilitation programs and back school for patients with low back pain: a meta-analysis. *Phys Ther.* 1995;75(10):865-878.

25. Clauser G. Back basics: teaching tips for a healthy back. *Physical Therapy Today.* 1995; 8-9, 12, 15.

26. Bulaclac MC. A work site wellness program. *Nursing Management.* 1996;27(12):19-21.

27. Pruitt RH. Effectiveness and cost efficiency of interventions in health promotion. *J Adv Nurs.* 1992;17:926-932.

28. Griffith HM. The costs of clinical prevention services. *J Prof Nurs.* 1994;10(6):331, 372.

29. Relfe S. Maintaining the independence of residents in retirement communities. *Geriatric Care and Rehabilitation.* 1995;9(6):1-8.

30. Molzahn AE. Changing to a caring paradigm for teaching and learning. *ANNA Journal.* 1996;23(1):13-18.

31. Davolt S. New niches in physical fitness. *PT-Magazine of Physical Therapy.* 1997;5(3):32-41.

32. Ellis J. Physical therapy interventions help performers prevent injuries. *PT Bulletin.* 1997;12(17):9.

33. Williams RB, Boles M, Jognson RE. Patient use of a computer for prevention in primary care practice. *Patient Education and Counseling.* 1995;(25):283-292.

34. New cyberspace clinic offers personalized weight-loss advice. *PT Bulletin.* 1996;11(45):1.

35. Internet brings two families together. *PT Bulletin.* 1997;12(10):12.

TEST YOUR SKILLS

1. Scenario:

You are the clinical director of an outpatient rehabilitation facility. At your clinic, a variety of patients are seen, and 85% of that population has secondary health complications that may or may not impact their improvement or progression. What types of primary, secondary, or tertiary preventative measures can you and your staff do?

Primary:

Secondary:

Tertiary:

2. You have developed a workplace wellness program you wish to market to computer companies. How will you convince a prospective client of the benefits of offering your program to their employees?

CHECK YOUR RESPONSES

1. Scenario:

Primary:
*   Weight control/management
*   Exercise classes/instruction
*   Pamphlets/information/classes available on several diseases, disorders, and preventative measures (ie, fall prevention, osteoporosis)

Secondary:
*   Back school for patients with back problems, including weakness, pain, and poor body mechanics
*   Postural exams/screenings
*   Work hardening for patients following a back injury prior to "return to work"
*   Balance evaluations for patients at possible risk for falls

Tertiary:
*   Aqua aerobics for patients with such debilitating conditions as rheumatoid arthritis, degenerative disk disease, multiple sclerosis, and polio
*   Splints made for patients with deformities to improve function, normalize tone, and prevent further limitations

2. Workplace wellness program proposal:

By investing in our program, your company will experience a substantial decrease in employee sick days and an increase in physical condition, health, strength, employee morale, and job performance.

Our company offers a wide variety of services that can be tailored to meet the needs of your company. The following are a few of the areas of focus we provide:
*   Injury consultation
*   Ergonomic improvement in workstations
*   Postural exams and biomechanical suggestions/training
*   Exercise and diet education
*   Computer equipment suggestions
*   General health promotion

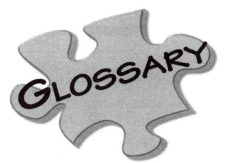

Accreditation An organization recognizes an institution as meeting predetermined standards.

Administrative costs Costs incurred by health care insurers relating, but not limited, to utilization review, insurance marketing, medical underwriting, agents' commissions, premium collection, claims processing, insurer profit, quality assurance programs, and risk management.

Adverse selection Among applicants for a given group or individual program, the tendency for those with an impaired health status, or who are prone to higher than average utilization of benefits, to be enrolled in disproportionate numbers and lower deductible plans.

Adjusted average per capita cost (AAPCC) The estimated average fee-for-service cost of Medicare benefits for an individual by county of residence. It is based on the following factors: age, sex, institutional status, Medicaid, disability, and end-stage renal disease status. Health Care Financing Administration uses the AAPCC as a basis for making monthly payments to Tax Equity and Fiscal Responsibility Act of 1992 (TEFRA) contractors.

Agency for Health Care Policy and Research (AHCPR) The agency of the Public Health Service responsible for enhancing the quality, appropriateness, and effectiveness of health care services. The agency was created by Congress in 1989 to engage in quality improvement-related activities, including development of peer-reviewed outcomes studies and practice parameters.

Ambulatory care Health care services provided on an outpatient basis. No overnight stay in a hospital is required. The services of ambulatory care centers, hospital outpatient departments, physicians' offices, and home health care services fall under this heading.

Ambulatory patient groups (APGs) A prospective payment system involving classification of individuals for outpatient care by diagnostic category and prior use of services in either inpatient or outpatient settings.

Average length of stay (ALOS) Refers to the average length of stay per inpatient hospital visit. Figure is typically calculated for both commercial and Medicare patient populations.

Balanced Budget Act of 1997 Legislation that provided cost containment in Medicare program; mandated a shift from fee-for-service to prospective payment system for long-term care facilities and capped therapy benefits under Medicare Part B reimbursement. Required implementation of prospective payment systems for patients in skilled nursing facilities covered by Medicare Part A (Resource Utilization Groups System III) and Medicare Part B (fee schedules).

Beneficiary Individual who is either using or eligible to use insurance benefits, including health insurance benefits, under an insurance contract.

Benefit payment schedule List of amounts an insurance plan will pay for covered health care services.

Benefits The payment for or health care services provided under terms of a contract with a managed care organization (MCO).

Capitation A payment system whereby managed care plans pay health care providers a fixed amount to care for a patient over a given period. Providers are not reimbursed for services that exceed the allotted amount. The rate may be fixed for all members, or it can be adjusted for the age and gender of the member, based on actuarial projections of medical utilization.

Carve-out arrangement The process of minimizing financial risk in a capitated contract by "carving out" or removing services over which a physician or other provider group has no control. Commonly carved-out services include behavioral health, laboratory, and x-ray services.

Cascading coverage A reimbursement plan used by workers' compensation administrators in which provider services are reimbursed at 100% of a set fee schedule for the first procedure and then at a diminishing rate of the fee schedule (ie, 75%, 50%, 25%, etc) for each additional procedure during an office visit.

Case management The process by which all health-related matters of a case are managed by a physician, nurse, or designated health professional. Physician case managers coordinate designated components of health care, such as appropriate referral to consultants, specialists, hospitals, ancillary providers, and services. Case management is intended to ensure continuity of services and accessibility to overcome rigidity, fragmented services, and the inappropriate utilization of facilities and resources. It also attempts to match the appropriate intensity of services with the patient's needs over time.

Case rate Flat fee paid for a client's treatment based on his or her diagnosis and/or presenting problem. For this fee, the provider covers all of the services the client requires for a specific period of time, also known as a bundled rate or flat fee per case. It is very often used as an intervening step prior to capitation. In this model, the provider is accepting some significant risk but does have considerable flexibility in how it meets the client's needs. Keys to success in this mode: 1. properly pricing a case rate, if the provider has control over it; and 2. securing a large volume of eligible clients.

CHAMPUS Civilian Health and Medical Program of the Uniformed Services.

Claims review The method by which an enrollee's health care service claims are reviewed prior to reimbursement. The purpose is to validate the medical necessity of the provided services and to be sure the cost of the service is not excessive.

Closed access A managed health care arrangement in which covered people are required to select providers only from the plan's participating providers.

Closed panel Medical services are delivered in the HMO-owned health center or satellite clinic by physicians who belong to a specially formed, but legally separate, medical group that only serves the HMO. This term generally applies only to staff and group model HMOs. This term may also be used to designate a physician practice that is closed to new patients.

Co-insurance A cost-sharing requirement under a health insurance policy that provides that the insured will assume a portion or percentage of the costs of covered services. After the deductible is paid, this provision forces the subscriber to pay for a certain percentage of any remaining medical bills, usually 20%.

Community rating Setting insurance rates based on the average cost of providing health services to all people in a geographic area, without adjusting for each individual's medical history or likelihood of using medical services.

Co-morbidity The presence of multiple diagnoses requiring management. For example, a patient might have an acute problem, such as surgical fixation of a hip fracture, but also have diabetes, renal disease, hypertension, and a history of breast cancer. These multiple problems require monitoring and may complicate or slow patient progress.

Concurrent review Review of a procedure or hospital admission done by a health care professional (usually a nurse) while the service is being performed. Concurrent review may be done off-site through the use of a telephone or fax, or at the site of care.

Coordination of benefits (COB) Provisions and procedures used by third-party payers to determine the amount payable to each payer when a claimant is covered under two or more group health plans.

Copayment A type of cost-sharing that requires the insured or subscriber to pay a specified flat dollar amount, usually on a per unit of service basis, with the third-party payer reimbursing some portion of remaining charges.

Cost sharing The general set of financing arrangements whereby the consumer must pay out-of-pocket to receive care, either at the time of initiating care, or during the provision of health care services, or both. Cost sharing can also occur when an insured pays a portion of the monthly premium for health care insurance.

Cost shifting Charging one group of patients more in order to make up for underpayment by others. Most commonly, charging some privately insured patients more in order to make up for underpayment by Medicaid or Medicare.

Credentialing The process of reviewing a practitioners' credentials, ie, training, experience, or demonstrated ability, for the purpose of determining if criteria for clinical privileges are met.

Clinical or critical pathways A "map" of preferred treatment/intervention activities. Outlines the types of information needed to make decisions, the timelines for applying that information, and what action needs to be taken by whom. Provides a way to monitor care "in real time." These pathways are developed by clinicians for specific diseases or events. Pro-active providers are working now to develop these pathways for the majority of their interventions and developing the software capacity to distribute and store this information.

Common procedural terminology (CPT) A uniform coding system for therapy services that is used to determine provider fee schedule reimbursement.

Concurrent review A routine review by an internal or external utilization reviewer during the course of a patient's treatment to determine if continued treatment is medically necessary. This usually occurs for inpatient, residential, and partial hospitalization treatment, though it is becoming more frequent for outpatient as well.

Days/1000/year A common utilization measurement used in the health care industry that refers to a ratio of the number of days a patient population has for a particular service, per 1,000 members enrolled for a given year. For example, if an HMO with 10,000 members experiences 3,800 total hospital days, the relevant ratio is 380 hospital days per 1,000 members per year.

Deductible The out-of-pocket expenses that must be borne by an insurance subscriber before the insurer will begin reimbursing the subscriber for additional expenses.

Diagnosis-related groups (DRG) A system used by Medicare and other insurers to classify illnesses according to diagnosis and treatment. All Medicare inpatient hospital operating costs are determined in advance and paid on a per-case basis, according to a fixed amount or weight established for each DRG.

Discounted fee-for-service An agreed-upon rate for service between the provider and payer that is usually less than the provider's full fee. This may be a fixed amount per service or a percentage discount. Providers generally accept such contracts because they represent a means to increase their volume or reduce their chances of losing volume.

Direct access The ability to treat clients needing physical therapy without the legal requirement of practitioner referral. Most states allow direct access for physical therapy evaluation. Many states allow direct access for physical therapy services for both evaluation and treatment.

Early and periodic screening, diagnosis, and treatment (EPSDT) An EPSDT program covers screening and diagnostic services to determine physical or mental defects in Medicaid recipients under age 21, as well as health care and other measures to correct or ameliorate any defects and chronic conditions discovered.

Employee Retirement Income Security Act (ERISA) A 1974 federal law that governs self-funded employer health benefit programs. ERISA exempts self-insured health plans from state laws governing health insurance, including contribution to risk pools, prohibitions against disease discrimination, and other state health reforms.

Enrollee Any person eligible, as either a subscriber or a dependent, in an employee benefit plan. (Synonyms: beneficiary, eligible individual, member, participant)

External quality review organization (EQRO) States are required to contract with an entity that is external to and independent of the state and its HMO contractors to perform an annual review of the quality of services furnished by each HMO.

Exclusions Clauses in a health insurance contract that deny coverage for select individuals, groups, locations, properties, or risks; clauses in a health insurance contract specifying which services/procedures are not available as a benefit.

Exclusive provider organization (EPO) A managed care organization that is organized similarly to a PPO in that physicians do not receive capitated payments, but that only allows patients to choose medical care from network providers. If a patient elects to seek care outside of the network, then he or she will not be reimbursed for the cost of the treatment.

Exclusivity clause A part of a contract that prohibits physicians from contracting with more than one managed care organization (HMO, PPO, IPA, etc).

Experience rating A process wherein insurance companies evaluate the risk of an individual or group by looking at the applicant's health history and utilization.

Federally qualified HMOs HMOs that meet certain federally stipulated provisions aimed at protecting consumers, eg, providing a broad range of basic health services, assuring financial solvency, and monitoring the quality of care. HMOs must apply to the federal government for qualification. The process is administered by the Health Care Financing Administration, Department of Health and Human Services.

Federal Medicaid managed care waiver program The process used by states to receive permission to implement managed care programs for their Medicaid or other categorically eligible beneficiaries.

Fee disclosure Physicians and caregivers discussing their charges with patients prior to treatment.

Fee for service (FFS) The traditional payment method whereby patients pay doctors, hospitals, and other providers for services rendered and then bill private insurers or the government.

Fee schedule A comprehensive listing of fees used by either a health care plan or the government to reimburse physicians and/or other providers on a fee-for-service basis.

Fiscal intermediary The agent (ie, Blue Cross) that has contracted with providers of service to process claims for reimbursement under health care coverage. In addition to handling financial matters, it may perform other functions, such as providing consultative services or serving as a center for communication with providers and making audits of providers' needs.

Flat fee per case Flat fee paid for a client's treatment based on his or her diagnosis and/or presenting problem. For this fee, the provider covers all of the services the client requires for a specific period of time. See case rate, above.

Formulary A list of selected pharmaceuticals and their appropriate dosages felt to be the most useful and cost effective for patient care. Organizations often develop a formulary under the aegis of a pharmacy and therapeutics committee. In HMOs, physicians are often required to prescribe from the formulary.

Function-related groups (FRGs) A prospective payment system that groups patients by their level of functional independence in an effort to take into account the volume and intensity of services required.

Gatekeeper A primary care physician responsible for overseeing and coordinating all aspects of a patient's medical care. For a patient to receive a specialty care referral or hospital admission, the gatekeeper must pre-authorize the visit, unless there is an emergency.

Group insurance Any insurance policy or health services contract by which groups of employees (and often their dependents) are covered under a single policy or contract issued by their employer or other group entity.

Group or network model HMO An HMO that contracts with a multispecialty medical group to provide care for HMO members; members are required to receive medical care from a physician within the group unless a referral is made outside the network.

Health Care Financing Administration (SCFA) Federal agency that administers the Medicare program.

Health Maintenance Organization (HMO) HMOs offer prepaid, comprehensive health coverage for both hospital and physician services. An HMO contracts with health care providers (ie, physicians, hospitals, and other health professionals), and members are required to use participating providers for all health services. Members are enrolled for a specified period of time. Model types include staff, group practice, network, and IPA (for additional information, see staff, group, network and independent practice association model definitions).

Health plan employer data and information set (HEDIS) A set of performance measures designed to standardize the way health plans report data to employers. HEDIS currently measures five major areas of health plan performance: quality, access and patient satisfaction, membership and utilization, finance, and descriptive information on health plan management.

Hold harmless clause A clause frequently found in managed care contracts whereby the HMO and the physician hold each other not liable for malpractice or corporate malfeasance if either of the parties is found to be liable. Many insurance carriers exclude this type of liability from coverage. It may also refer to language that prohibits the provider from billing patients if its managed care company becomes insolvent. State and federal regulations may require this language.

Home health agencies Public or private agencies or organizations primarily engaged in providing skilled nursing or other therapeutic services in the home.[5]

Home health care Health and social services delivered in the homes of recovering, disabled, or chronically or terminally ill people in need of medical, nursing, social, or therapeutic treatment and/or assistance with the essential activities of daily living. Home care also includes the provision of equipment and services to the patient in the home for the purposes of restoring and maintaining their maximal level of comfort, function, safety, and health.

Hospice care Hospice care involves an interdisciplinary team of health care providers and volunteers who provide medical care, as well as psychological and spiritual care, for the terminally ill. They also provide support for the patients' families. Hospice services are available to individuals who are terminally ill and have a life expectancy of 6 months or less. Services are generally covered under Medicare. Care includes the provision of related medications, medical supplies, and equipment. It is based primarily in the home, allowing families to stay together.

Indemnify To make good on a loss.

Indemnity health insurance A traditional health insurance plan with little or no benefit management, a fee-for-service reimbursement model, and few restrictions on provider selection. Generally no longer in existence.

Independent practice association (IPA) A health maintenance organization delivery model in which the HMO contracts with a physician organization that, in turn, contracts with individual physicians. The IPA physicians practice in their own offices and continue to see fee-for-service patients. The HMO reimburses the IPA on a capitated basis; however, the IPA usually reimburses the physicians on a fee-for-service basis. This type of system combines prepayment with the traditional means of delivering health care.

Inpatient services Inpatient hospital services are items and services furnished to a hospital inpatient by the hospital, including bed and board, nursing and related services, diagnostic and therapeutic services, and medical or surgical services.

Licensing A process most states employ, which involves the review and approval of applications from HMOs prior to beginning operation in certain areas of the state. Areas examined by the licensing authority include fiscal soundness, network capacity, management information systems (MIS), and quality assurance. The applicant must demonstrate it can meet all existing statutory and regulatory requirements prior to beginning operations.

Long-term care facility A residential facility that offers custodial care to residents unable to care for themselves and who do not have family members capable of caring for them.

Managed care A general term for organizing physicians, hospitals, and other providers into groups in order to enhance the quality and cost effectiveness of health care. Managed care organizations include HMOs, PPOs, POSs, EPOs, etc. This arrangement integrates financing and management with the delivery of health care services to an enrolled population. It employs or contracts with an organized system of providers that delivers services and frequently shares financial risk.

Managed services organization (MSO) An entity that contracts for the provision of management and administrative support services to health care providers, including physicians and physician networks. Usually organized by a hospital, services offered through an MSO may include (among others) claims processing, billing and collection services, personnel recruitment, group purchasing, information management systems, contract negotiations and administration, utilization review, quality assurance, and credentialing.

Market share That proportion of eligible enrollees in a defined market that a managed care or insurance company has enrolled as members in its plan; usually market share is expressed as a percentage of the market potential.

Medical group practice The American Group Practice Association, the American Medical Association, and the Medical Group Management Association define medical group practice as, "provision of health care services by a group of at least three licensed physicians engaged in a formally organized and legally recognized entity sharing equipment, facilities, common records, and personnel involved in both patient care and business management."

Medical savings account (MSA) An employment-based health insurance plan in which employers purchase less expensive health plans with high deductibles for employees who choose to participate. The annual price difference between the highest priced health plan offered and the cheaper health plan purchased is put into a medical savings account for the employee.

Medically necessary Those covered services required to preserve and maintain the health status of a member or eligible person in accordance with the area standards of medical practice. They generally meet the following tests: they are appropriate and necessary for the symptoms, diagnosis, or treatment of the medical condition; they are provided for the diagnosis or direct care and treatment of the medical condition; they meet the standards of good medical practice within the medical community in the service area; they are not primarily for the convenience of the plan member or a plan provider; and they are the most appropriate level or supply of service that can safely be provided. This standard is becoming the most important one for providers to focus on.

Medicare supplement policy A health insurance policy that pays certain costs not covered by Medicare, such as coinsurance and deductibles.

Multispecialty group A group of doctors who represent various medical specialties and who work together in a group practice.

Multi-skilled workers A label referring to nonprofessional support personnel who have been cross-trained in areas of practice in which the individual is neither educated nor licensed. These workers provide a variety of technical services in health care delivery. For example, a worker might provide for routine daily patient care needs supervised by nursing and physical therapy. Titles for these workers vary; some facilities call them service associates, care partners, care associates, and technical partners.

National Committee for Quality Assurance (NCQA) A nonprofit organization created to improve patient care quality and health plan performance in partnership with managed care plans, purchasers, consumers, and the public sector.

Network model HMO An HMO that contracts with two or more independent group practices to provide health services. This type may include a few solo practices but is primarily organized around groups.

Open enrollment A period of time in which eligible subscribers may elect to enroll,or transfer between available programs providing health care coverage.

Outcomes Management A technology of patient experience designed to help patients, payers, and providers make more rational medical care-related choices based on better insight into the effect of these choices on the patient's life. Through longitudinal observational studies, outcomes management seeks to measure and evaluate a patient's functional health status and quality of life over time and to document changes in the patient's clinical condition as a result of therapeutic interventions. Outcomes management differs from clinical trials in that data are collected as part of routine medical care, and it attempts to determine what is appropriate resource consumption.

Out-of-area benefits Benefits supplied by a plan to its subscribers or enrollees when they need services outside the geographic limits of the HMO. These benefits usually include emergency care benefits, plus low fee-for-service payments for non-emergency care.

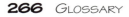

Outlier One who does not fall within the norm; term typically used in utilization review. A provider who uses either too many or too few services (for example, anyone whose utilization differs two standard deviations from the mean on a bell curve is termed an *outlier*).

Outpatient services Outpatient services are medical and other services provided by a hospital or other qualified facility, such as a mental health clinic, rural health clinic, mobile x-ray unit, or free-standing dialysis unit. Such services include outpatient physical therapy services, diagnostic x-ray, and laboratory tests.

Participating provider A health care provider who participates through a contractual arrangement with a health care service contractor, HMO, PPO, IPA, or other managed care organization.

Patient-focused care The organization and delivery of services in such a way that the patient's needs and cost containment are maximized. Involves decentralization of services, training of multi-skilled (technical) personnel, and development of critical pathways.

Primary care case management (PCCM) A PCCM program is a Freedom of Choice Waiver program, under the authority of section 1915(b) of the Social Security Act. States contract directly with primary care providers who agree to be responsible for the provision and/or coordination of medical services to Medicaid recipients under their care. Currently, most PCCM programs pay the primary care physician a monthly case management fee in addition to receiving fee-for-services payment.

Peer review A review by members of the same profession (peers) regarding the quality of care provided to a patient, including documentation of care (medical audit), diagnostic steps used, conclusions reached, therapy given, appropriateness of utilization (utilization review), and reasonableness of charges and claims.

Peer review organization (PRO) An organization established by the Tax Equity and Fiscal Responsibility Act of 1982 to review quality of care and appropriateness of admissions, re-admissions, and discharges for Medicare and Medicaid.

Performance standards Standards an individual provider is expected to meet, especially with respect to quality of care. The standards may define volume of care delivered per time period. Thus, performance standards for an obstetrician/gynecologist may specify some or all of the following office hours and office visits per week or month, on-call days, deliveries per year, gynecological operations per year, etc.

Physical therapist assistant An educated health care provider who assists the physical therapist in providing physical therapy by performing physical therapy procedures and related tasks that have been selected and delegated by the supervising physical therapist.

Physical therapy The care and services provided by or under the direction and supervision of a *physical therapist*. Defined as the assessment, evaluation, treatment, and prevention of physical disability, movement dysfunction, and pain resulting from injury, disease, disability, or other health-related conditions. Includes interpretation of referrals when available; initial examination; problem identification; evaluation; diagnosis; development of a plan of care; prognosis; application and/or supervision of physical therapy interventions/ treatment; timely review of treatment documentation; re-examination of the patient and the patient's treatment goals; revision of the plan of care when indicated; establishment of the discharge plan; and documentation of discharge summary or status. Only selected interventions may be delegated to physical therapy support personnel.

Physical therapy aide A nonlicensed worker who is specifically trained under the direction of a physical therapist and performs designated routine tasks related to the operation of a physical therapy service.

Physical therapist support personnel Physical therapist assistants, physical therapy aides, and others who work under the direction of physical therapists.

Per member per month (PMPM) The average cost of providing services to any member per month.

Point-of-service (POS) plan Also known as an open-ended HMO, POS plans encourage, but do not require, members to choose a primary care physician. As in traditional HMOs, the primary care physician acts as a "gatekeeper" when making referrals; plan members may, however, opt to visit non-network providers at their discretion. Subscribers choosing not to use the primary care physician must pay higher deductibles and copays than those using network physicians.

Practice parameters The American Medical Association defines practice parameters as strategies for patient management developed to assist physicians in clinical decision making. Practice parameters may also refer to practice options, practice guidelines, practice policies, or practice standards.

Practice profiling Analysis and summary of data to show provider outcomes and costs in relationship to those of other providers (for example, hospitals that have a higher than average readmission rate).

Pre-admission review The practice of reviewing claims for inpatient admission prior to the patient entering the hospital in order to ensure that the admission is medically necessary.

Pre-authorization A method of monitoring and controlling utilization by evaluating the need for medical service prior to it being performed.

Pre-certification The prior authorization required by some payers before health benefit payments will be authorized.

Pre-determination An administrative procedure whereby a health provider submits a treatment plan to a third party before treatment is initiated. The third party usually reviews the treatment plan, monitoring one or more of the following: patient's eligibility, covered service, amounts payable, application of appropriate deductibles, copayment factors, and maximums. Under some programs, for instance, pre-determination by the third party is required when covered charges are expected to exceed a certain amount. Similar processes: pre-authorization, pre-certification, pre-estimate of cost, pretreatment estimate, prior authorization.

Preferred provider organization (PPO) A health care arrangement between purchasers of care (ie, employers, insurance companies) and providers that offers benefits at a reasonable cost by providing member incentives (such as lower deductibles and copays) to use providers within the network. Members who prefer to use non-preferred physicians may do so, but only at a higher cost. Preferred providers must agree to specified fee schedules in exchange for a preferred status and are required to comply with certain utilization review guidelines.

Premium Money paid out in advance for insurance coverage.

Prepayment A method of paying for the cost of health care services in advance of their use.

Preventive health care Health care that seeks to prevent or foster early detection of disease and morbidity and focuses on keeping patients well in addition to helping them while they are sick.

Primary care The provision of integrated, accessible health care services by clinicians who are accountable for addressing a large majority of personal health care needs, developing a sustained partnership with patients, and practicing in the context of family and community.

Primary care network (PCN) A group of primary care physicians who share the risk of providing care to members of a given health plan.

Primary care provider (PCP) The provider that serves as the initial interface between the member and the medical care system. The PCP is usually a physician, selected by the member upon enrollment, who is trained in one of the primary care specialties, and who treats and is responsible for coordinating the treatment of members assigned to his or her plan (see also gatekeeper).

Professional review organization An organization that reviews the services provided to patients in terms of medical necessity, professional standards, and appropriateness of setting.

Profile Aggregated data in formats that display patterns of health care services over a defined period of time.

Quality assurance (QA), Quality Management (QM), Continuous Quality Improvement (CQI) Activities and programs intended to ensure the quality of care in a defined medical setting. Such programs include peer or utilization review components to identify and remedy deficiencies in quality. The program must have a mechanism for assessing its effectiveness and may measure care against pre-established standards.

Quality Assurance Reform Initiative (QARI) The Quality Assurance Reform Initiative was unveiled in 1993 to assist states in the development of continuous quality improvement systems, external quality assurance programs, internal quality assurance programs, and focused clinical studies.

Risk The chance or possibility of loss. For example, physicians may be held at risk if hospitalization rates exceed agreed-upon thresholds. The sharing of risk is often employed as a utilization control mechanism within the HMO setting. Risk is also defined in insurance terms as the possibility of loss associated with a given population.

Resource-based relative value scale (RBRVS) A Medicare weighting system to assign units of value to each CPT code (procedure) performed by physicians and other providers. The number of units or value for each procedure includes a portion for physician skill, expenses associated with the procedure, and geographic area. Loved by "process" doctors, such as PCPs, because adoption of this scale by Medicare increased their pay; despised by "transaction" doctors, such as specialists and surgeons, because they lost money per transaction.

Retrospective review process A review that is conducted after services are provided to a patient. The review focuses on determining the appropriateness, necessity, quality, and reasonableness of health care services provided. It is becoming the least desirable method, supplanted by concurrent reviews.

Risk adjustment A system of adjusting rates paid to managed care providers to account for the differences in beneficiary demographics, such as age, gender, race, ethnicity, medical condition, geographic location, at-risk population (ie, homeless), etc.

Risk pool A pool of money that is to be used for defined expenses. Commonly, if the money that is put at risk is not expended by the end of the year, some or all of it is returned to those managing the risk.

Risk sharing A method by which medical insurance premiums are shared by plan sponsors and participants. In contrast to traditional indemnity plans in which insurance premiums belonged solely to insurance companies that assumed all risk of using these premiums. The key to this approach is that the premiums are the only payment providers receive; it provides powerful incentive to limit services provided.

Resource utilization groups system (RUGS III) A classification system associated with the implementation of a prospective payment system for patients in skilled nursing facilities covered by Medicare Part A. The system identifies the relative costs of patient care based on the type of services and resources provided (Balanced Budget Act of 1997).

Self-insurance The practice of an employer or organization assuming responsibility for health care losses of its employees. This usually includes setting up a fund against which claim payments are drawn. Claims processing is often handled through an administrative services contract with an independent organization.

Shared savings A provision of most prepaid health care plans in which at least part of the provider's income is directly linked to the financial performance of the plan. If costs are lower than projections, a percentage of these savings are referred to the providers.

Skilled nursing facility (SNF) A facility offering sub-acute level of care meeting Medicare requirements for staffing and types of services offered.

Staff model HMO An HMO that delivers health services through a physician group that is controlled by the HMO unit; most physicians are salaried employees who deal exclusively with HMO members.

Tax equity and fiscal responsibility Act of 1982 (TEFRA) The federal law that created the current risk and cost contract provisions under which health plans contract with HCFA.

Tertiary care Subspecialty care usually requiring the facilities of a university-affiliated or teaching hospital that has extensive diagnostic and treatment capabilities.

Third-party administrator or third-party payer Individual or company that contracts with employers who want to self-insure the health of their employees. They develop and coordinate self-insurance programs, process and pay the claim, and may help locate stop-loss insurance for the employer. They also can analyze the effectiveness of the program and trace the patterns of those using the benefits.

Treatment episode The period of treatment between admission and discharge from a modality, (ie, inpatient, residential, partial hospitalization, and outpatient). Many health care statistics and profiles use this unit as abase for comparisons.

Usual, customary, and reasonable (UCR) A reimbursement method whereby a health insurance plan pays a physician's full charge if it is reasonable and does not exceed his or her usual charges and the amount customarily charged for the service by other physicians in the area.

Utilization The patterns of use of a service or type of service within a specified time. Utilization is usually expressed in rate per unit of population-at-risk for a given period (eg, the number of hospital admissions per year per 1,000 people enrolled in an HMO).

Utilization review (UR) A systematic means for reviewing and controlling patients' use of medical care services as well as the appropriateness and quality of that care. Usually involves data collection, review, and/or authorization, especially for services such as specialist referrals, emergency room use, and hospitalization.

Utilization management (UM) The process of evaluating the necessity, appropriateness, and efficiency of health care services against established guidelines and criteria.

Withhold That portion of the monthly reimbursement to physicians withheld by an HMO to create an incentive for efficient care. A physician who exceeds utilization norms does not receive the withheld amount. This system serves as a financial incentive for lower utilization. The withhold can cover all services or be specific to hospital care, laboratory usage, or specialty referrals.

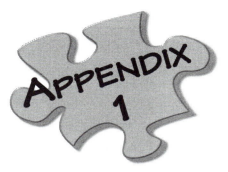

COMMONLY APPROVED PHYSICAL THERAPY ABBREVIATIONS

Abbreviations

AAROM	active assisted range of motion
abd.	abduction
add.	adduction
ADL	activities of daily living
AFO	ankle foot orthosis
A/K Amp	above-knee amputation
A.M.	morning
AODM	adult-onset diabetes mellitus
approx	approximately
ARDS	adult respiratory distress syndrome
AROM	active range of motion
ASAP	as soon as possible
b.i.d.	twice daily
BLE	both lower extremities
B.M.	bowel movement
BUE	both upper extremities
c	with
CABG	coronary artery bypass graft
CCS	California Children Services
CCU	coronary care unit
CHF	congestive heart failure
CNS	central nervous system
c/o	complains of
cont	continue
COPD	chronic obstructive pulmonary disease
CP	cerebral palsy
c.r.	contract-relax
CSF	cerebral spinal fluid
CVA	cerebral vascular accident
dc	discontinued
D/C	discharged
DIP	distal interphalangeal joint
DNKA	did not keep appointment
Dr	doctor
dsg.	dressing
DTR	deep tendon reflex
DVT	deep venous thrombosis
DX	diagnosis
ECF	extended care facility
EKG/ECG	electrocardiogram
EMG	electromyogram or myograph
ER	emergency room

ES	electrical stimulation	KAFO	knee, ankle, foot orthosis
etc	and so on	L	left
ETOH	alcohol	lat	lateral
ext rot	external rotation	lat. bar.	latissimus dorsi bar
flex/ext	flexion extension	lb	pound
ft	feet	LBP	low back pain
FWB	full weight bearing	LE	lower extremity
FWW	front wheeled walker	lg	large
GCS	Glasgow Coma Scale	LLB	long leg brace
GSH	gun shot wound	LLC	long leg cast
HA	headache	LLE	left lower extremity
HAb/HAd	horizontal abduction/ adduction	LLL	left lower lobe
		LOB	loss of balance
hams	hamstrings	LOC	loss of consciousness
HBP	high blood pressure	LP	lumbar puncture
hemi	hemiplegia	LUE	left upper extremity
HNP	herniated nucleus pulposus	LUL	left upper lobe
H/O	history of	max	maximum
HOB	head of bed	MC	metacarpal
H.P.	hot pack	MCA	motorcycle accident
hr	hour	MCP	metacarpalphalangeal
HR	heart rate	M.D.	muscular dystrophy
HT	hubbard tank	M.I.	myocardial infarct
HTN	hypertension	MICU	medical intensive care unit
Hx	history	min	minute
ICP	intracranial pressure	MMT	manual muscle test
ICT	intermittent cervical traction	mod	moderate
		MP	metacarpal-phalangeal
I&D	incision and drainage	MRE	manual resistive exercise
IDDM	insulin-dependent diabetes mellitus	MTP	metatarsophalangeal
		MVA	motor vehicle accident
inv/ev	inversion/eversion	N	normal
IP	interphalangeal	N.	nerve
IPTX	intermittent pelvic traction	N/A	not applicable
IV	intravenous	NDT	neurodevelopmental treatment
JOMACI	judgment, orientation, memory, abstraction, and calculation		
		neg	negative
		neurosurg.	neurosurgery
Jt	joint	NIDDM	non insulin-dependent diabetes mellitus
JW	jumpwalker		

NWB	non-weight bearing		quad	quadriplegia
0	none		quads	quadriceps
O_2	oxygen		R	right
obs	observation		RAM	rapid alternating movements
OOB	out of bed		reps	repetitions
O.P.	outpatient		RLE	right lower extremity
o.p.	overpressure		RLL	right lower lobe
OR	operating room		RM	repeated movements
ORIF	open reduction internal fixation		RN	registered nurse
ortho	orthopedics		R/O	rule out
OT	occupational therapy		ROM	range of motion
O x 3	oriented to person, place, and time		RUE	right upper extremity
			Rx	treatment
p	after or post		S	supervision
P-A	posterior-anterior		SAC	short arm cast
Para	paraplegic		SAQ	short arc quads
P/D flex	plantar flexion/dorsiflexion		SBA	stand by assist
PE	pulmonary embolism		SCI	spinal cord injury
peds	pediatrics		SCTx	static cervical traction
PICU	pediatric intensive care unit		sec.	second
PIJ	proximal interphalangeal joint		sh	shoulder
			SICU	surgical intensive care unit
P.M.	afternoon		SLB	short leg brace
PNF	proprioceptive neuro-muscular facilitation		sld. bd.	sliding board
			SLR	straight leg raise
PRE	passive resistive exercises		SLWC	short leg walking cast
prn	whenever necessary		SOAP	subjective/objective/assessment/plan
PROM	passive range of motion			
prox	proximal		SOB	shortness of breath
psych	psychiatry		S/P	status post
pt	patient		SPTx	static pelvic traction
PT	physical therapy		S.T.	speech therapy
PTA	prior to admission		stat	immediately
PTB cast	patellar tendon bearing cast		STSG	split thickness skin graft
PTB prosth	patellar tendon bearing prosthesis		sup	superior
			surg	surgery
PUW	pick up walker		Sx	symptoms
PWB	partial weight bearing		T	temperature
q	every		TBI	traumatic brain injury
QEE	quadriceps extension exercises		TBSA	total body surface area

TDWB	touch down weight bearing
temp	temperature
TENS	transcutaneous electrical nerve stimulation
THR	total hip replacement
TIA	transient ischemic attack
TKR	total knee replacement
TLSO	thoracic lumbar sacral orthosis
TMJ	temperomandibular joint
TT	tilt table
Tx	treatment
UE	upper extremity
US	ultrasound
UTI	urinary tract infection
UV	ultraviolet
w.b.	weight bearing
w/c	wheelchair
WFL	within functional limits
WHO	wrist hand orthosis
wk.	week
WNL	within normal limits
WP	whirlpool
wt	weight
w/u	work up
x	times
y.o.	year old

Symbols

–	negative	2	secondary
+	positive	c	with
R	right	s	without
L	left	♀ ♂	female/male
#	pounds	> <	greater than/less than
I	independent	((	increase/decrease
@	at	//	parallel bars
B	both, bilateral	ᴈ	rotation
1	primary	4xd	four times a day

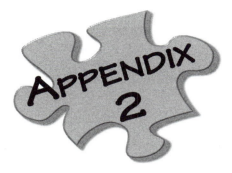

APTA GUIDELINES FOR PHYSICAL THERAPY DOCUMENTATION

The following is reprinted from APTA. *Guidelines for Physical Therapy Documentation*, with permission from the American Physical Therapy Association.

Guidelines for Physical Therapy Documentation

PREAMBLE

The American Physical Therapy Association (APTA) is committed to meeting the physical therapy needs of society, to meeting the needs and interests of its members, and to developing and improving the art and science of physical therapy, including practice, education, and research. To help meet these responsibilities, the APTA Board of Directors has approved the following guidelines for physical therapy documentation. It is recognized that these guidelines do not reflect all of the unique documentation requirements associated with the many specialty areas within the physical therapy profession. Applicable for both handwritten and electronic documentation systems, these guidelines are intended to be used as a foundation for the development of more specific documentation guidelines in specialty areas, while at the same time providing guidance for the physical therapy profession across all practice settings.

OPERATIONAL DEFINITIONS

Guidelines:

APTA defines "guidelines" as approved, non-binding statements of advice.

Documentation:

Any entry into the client record, such as: consultation report, initial examination report, progress note, flow sheet/checklist that identifies the care/service provided, reexamination, or summation of care.

Authentication:

The process used to verify that an entry is complete, accurate, and final. Indications of authentication can include original written signatures and computer "signatures" on secured electronic record systems only.

I. GENERAL GUIDELINES

A. All documentation must comply with the applicable jurisdictional/regulatory requirements.

1. All handwritten entries shall be made in ink and will include original signatures. Electronic entries should be made with appropriate security and confidentiality provisions.

2. Informed consent: As required by the APTA *Standards of Practice for Physical Therapy and the Accompanying Criteria*

2.1 The physical therapist has sole responsibility for providing information to the patient and for obtaining the patient's informed consent in accordance with jurisdictional law before initiating physical therapy.

2.2 Those deemed competent to give consent are competent adults. When the adult is not competent, and in the case of minors, a parent or legal guardian consents as the surrogate decision maker.

2.3 The information provided to the patient should include the following: (a) a clear description of the treatment ordered or recommended, (b) material (decisional) risks associated with the proposed treatment, (c) expected benefits of treatment, (d) comparison of the benefits and risks possible with and without treatment, and (e) reasonable alternatives to the recommended treatment. The physical therapist should solicit questions from the patient and provide answers. The patient should be asked to acknowledge understanding and consent before treatment proceeds.

Examples of ways in which to accomplish this documentation:

Ex 2.3.1 Signature of patient/ guardian on long or short consent form.

Ex 2.3.2 Notation/entry of what was explained by the physical therapist or the physical therapist assistant in the official record.

Ex 2.3.3 Filing of a completed consent checklist signed by the patient.

3. Charting errors should be corrected by drawing a single line through the error and initialing and dating the chart or through the appropriate mechanism for electronic documentation that clearly indicates that a change was made without deletion of the original record.

4. Identification.

4.1 Include patient's full name and identification number, if applicable, on all official documents.

4.2 All entries must be dated and authenticated with the provider's full name and appropriate designation (eg, PT, PTA).

4.3 Documentation by students (SPT/SPTA) shall be authenticated by a licensed physical therapist.

4.4 Documentation by graduates (GPT/GPTA) or others pending receipt of an unrestricted license shall be authenticated by a licensed physical therapist.

5. Documentation should include the manner in which physical therapy services are initiated.

Examples include:

Ex 5.1 Self-referral/direct access.

Ex 5.2 Attachment of the referral/consultation request by a qualified practitioner.

Ex 5.3 File copy of correspondence to referral source as acknowledgment of the referral.

II. INITIAL EXAMINATION AND EVALUATION/CONSULTATION

A. Documentation is required at the outset of each episode of physical therapy care.

B. Elements include:

1. Obtaining a history and identifying risk factors:

    1.1 History of the presenting problem, current complaints, and precautions (including onset date).

    1.2 Pertinent diagnoses and medical history.

    1.3 Demographic characteristics, including pertinent psychological, social, and environmental factors.

    1.4 Prior or concurrent services related to the current episode of physical therapy care.

    1.5 Comorbidities that may affect goals and treatment plan.

    1.6 Statement of patient's knowledge of problem.

    1.7 Goals of patient (and family members, or significant others, if appropriate).

2. Selecting and administering tests and measures to determine patient status in a number of areas. The following is a partial list of these areas, with illustrative tests and measures:

    2.1 Arousal, mentation, and cognition

    Examples include objective findings related, but not limited, to the following areas:

    > Ex 2.1.1 Level of consciousness
    > Ex 2.1.2 Ability to process commands
    > Ex 2.1.3 Alertness
    > Ex 2.1.4 Gross expressive and receptive language deficits

    2.2 Neuromotor development and sensory integration

    Examples include objective findings related, but not limited, to the following areas:

    > Ex 2.2.1 Gross and fine motor skills
    > Ex 2.2.2 Reflex and movement patterns
    > Ex 2.2.3 Dexterity, agility, and coordination

    2.3 Range of motion

    Examples include objective findings related, but not limited, to the following areas:

    > Ex 2.3.1 Extent of joint motion
    > Ex 2.3.1 Pain and soreness of surrounding soft tissue
    > Ex 2.3.2 Muscle length and flexibility

    2.4 Muscle performance

    Examples include objective findings related, but not limited, to the following areas:

    > Ex 2.4.1 Strength
    > Ex 2.4.2 Power
    > Ex 2.4.3 Endurance

    2.5 Ventilation, respiration, and circulation

    Examples include objective findings related, but not limited, to the following areas:

    > Ex 2.5.1 Vital signs
    > Ex 2.5.2 Breathing patterns
    > Ex 2.5.3 Heart sounds

    2.6 Posture

    Examples include objective findings related, but not limited, to the following areas:

    > Ex 2.6.1 Static posture
    > Ex 2.6.2 Dynamic posture

    2.7 Gait, locomotion, and balance

    Examples include objective findings related, but not limited, to the following areas:

    > Ex 2.7.1 Characteristics of gait
    > Ex 2.7.2 Functional ambulation
    > Ex 2.7.3 Characteristics of balance

    2.8 Self-care and home management status

    Examples include objective findings related, but not limited, to the following areas:

    > Ex 2.8.1 Activities of daily living
    > Ex 2.8.2 Functional capacity
    > Ex 2.8.3 Static and dynamic strength

    2.9 Community and work (job/school/play) integration/reintegration.

    > Ex 2.9.1 Instrumental activities of daily living
    > Ex 2.9.3 Functional capacity
    > Ex 2.9.3 Adaptive skills

3. Evaluation (a dynamic process in which the physical therapist makes clinical judgments based on data gathered during the examination).

4. Diagnosis (a label encompassing a cluster of signs and symptoms, syndromes, or categories that reflects the information obtained from the examination).

5. Goals.

    5.1 Patient (and family members or significant others, if appropriate) is involved in establishing goals.

    5.2 All goals are stated in measurable terms.

    5.3 Goals are linked to problems identified in the examination.

    5.4 Short- and long-term goals are established when applicable (may include potential for achieving goals).

6. Intervention plan or recommendation requirements:

    6.1 Shall be related to realistic goals and expected functional outcomes.

    6.2 Should include frequency and duration to achieve the stated goals.

    6.3 Should include patient and family/caregiver educational goals.

    6.4 Should involve appropriate collaboration and coordination of care with other professionals/services.

7. Authentication and appropriate designation of physical therapist.

III. DOCUMENTATION OF THE CONTINUUM OF CARE

A. Intervention or service provided.
1. Documentation is required for each patient visit/ encounter. Authentication is required for every note by the physical therapist or the physical therapist assistant providing the service under the supervision of the physical therapist.

   Examples include:

   Ex 1.1 Checklist
   Ex 1.2 Flow sheet
   Ex 1.3 Graph
   Ex 1.4 Narrative

2. Elements may include:

   2.1 Identification of specific interventions provided.
   2.2 Equipment provided.

B. Patient status, progress, or regression.
1. Documentation is required for every visit/encounter. Authentication is required for every note by the physical therapist or the physical therapist assistant providing the service under the supervision of the physical therapist.
2. Elements may include:

   2.1 Subjective status of patient.
   2.2 Changes in objective and measurable findings as they relate to existing goals.
   2.3 Adverse reaction to treatment.
   2.4 Progression/regression of existing therapeutic regimen, including patient education and adherence.
   2.5 Communication/consultation with providers/ patient/family/significant other.
   2.6 Authentication and appropriate designation of either a physical therapist or a physical therapist assistant.

C. Reexamination and Reevaluation
1. Documentation is required monthly for patients seen at intervals of a month of less; if the patient is seen less frequently, documentation is required for every visit or encounter.
2. Elements include:

   2.1 Documentation of elements as identified in III.B.2.1 through III.B.2.5 to update patient's status.
   2.2 Interpretation of findings and, when indicated, revision of goals.
   2.3 When indicated, revision of treatment plan, as directly correlated with documented goals.
   2.4 Authentication and appropriate designation of physical therapist.

IV. SUMMATION OF CARE

A. Documentation is required following conclusion of the current episode in the physical therapy care sequence.
B. Elements include:
1. Reason for discontinuation of service.

   Examples include:

   Ex 1.1 Satisfactory goal achievement.
   Ex 1.2 Patient declines to continue care.
   Ex 1.3 Patient is unable to continue to work toward goals due to medical or psychosocial complications.

2. Current physical/functional status.
3. Degree of goal achievement and reasons for goals not being achieved.
4. Discharge plan that includes written and verbal communication related to the patient's continuing care.

   Examples include:

   Ex 4.1 Home program.
   Ex 4.2 Referrals for additional services.
   Ex 4.3 Recommendations for follow-up physical therapy care.
   Ex 4.4 Family and caregiver training.
   Ex 4.5 Equipment provided.

5. Authentication and appropriate designation of physical therapist.

References

1. *Direction, Delegation and Supervision in Physical Therapy Services.* HOD 06-96-30-4)

2. *Comprehensive Accreditation Manual for Hospitals.* Oakbrook Terrace, Ill: Joint Commission on Accreditation of Healthcare Organizations; 1996.

3. *Glossary of Terms Related to Information Security.* Schamburg, Ill: Computer-Based Patient Record Institute; 1996

4. *Guidelines for Establishing Information Security Policies at Organizations Using Computer-Based Patient Records.* Schamburg, Ill: Computer-Based Patient Record Institute; 1995.

Adopted by the Board of Directors
March 1997
Amended March 1993, June 1993, November 1994, March 1995, March 1997

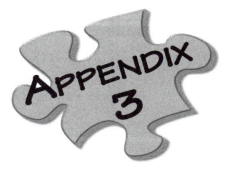

APPENDIX 3

APTA
STANDARDS OF PRACTICE

The following is reprinted from APTA. *Standards of Practice*, with permission from the American Physical Therapy Association.

●

Standards of Practice for Physical Therapy and the Accompanying Criteria

The Standards of Practice for Physical Therapy are promulgated by APTA's House of Delegates; the Criteria for the Standards are promulgated by APTA's Board of Directors. The Criteria are italicized beneath the Standards to which they apply.

PREAMBLE

The physical therapy profession is committed to providing an optimum level of service delivery and to striving for excellence in practice. The House of Delegates of the American Physical Therapy Association, as the formal body that represents the profession, attests to this commitment by adopting and promoting the following *Standards of Practice for Physical Therapy*. These *Standards of Practice for Physical Therapy* are the profession's statement of conditions and performances that are essential for provision of high-quality physical therapy. The *Standards* provide a foundation for assessment of physical therapy practice.

I. LEGAL/ETHICAL CONSIDERATIONS

A. Legal Considerations

The physical therapist complies with all the legal requirements of jurisdictions regulating the practice of physical therapy.

The physical therapist assistant complies with all the legal requirements of jurisdictions regulating the work of the assistant.

B. Ethical Considerations

The physical therapist practices according to the *Code of Ethics* of the American Physical Therapy Association.

The physical therapist assistant complies with the *Standards of Ethical Conduct for the Physical Therapist Assistant* of the American Physical Therapy Association.

II. ADMINISTRATION OF THE PHYSICAL THERAPY SERVICE

A. Statement of Mission, Purposes, and Goals

The physical therapy service has a statement of mission, purposes, and goals that reflects the needs and interests of the individuals served, the physical therapy personnel affiliated with the service, and the community.

Criteria
The statement:
- *Defines the scope and limitations of the service.*
- *Lists the goals and objectives of the service.*
- *Is reviewed annually.*

B. Organizational Plan

The physical therapy service has a written organizational plan.

Criteria
The plan:
- *Describes relationships within the service and, where the physical therapy service is part of a larger organization, between the physical therapy service and other components of the organization.*
- *Ensures that the service is directed by a physical therapist.*
- *Defines supervisory structures within the service.*
- *Reflects current personnel functions.*

C. Policies and Procedures

The physical therapy service has written policies and procedures that reflect the operation of the service and that are consistent with the mission, purposes, and goals of the service.

Criteria
The policies and procedures, which are reviewed regularly and revised as necessary, address pertinent information including (but not limited to) the following:
- *Clinical education.*
- *Clinical research.*
- *Interdisciplinary collaboration.*
- *Criteria for access to, initiation of, continuation of, referral of, and termination of care.*
- *Equipment maintenance.*
- *Environmental safety.*
- *Fiscal management.*
- *Infection control.*
- *Job/position descriptions.*
- *Competency assessment.*

- *Medical emergencies.*
- *Patient/client care policies and protocols.*
- *Patient/client rights.*
- *Personnel-related policies.*
- *Quality/performance improvement.*
- *Documentation.*
- *Staff orientation.*

The policies and procedures meet the requirements of state law and external agencies.

D. Administration
A physical therapist is responsible for the direction of the physical therapy service.

Criteria
The director:
- *Ensures compliance with local, state, and federal requirements.*
- *Ensures compliance with current APTA documents, including Standards of Practice for Physical Therapy, Guide for Professional Conduct, and Guide for Conduct of the Affiliate Member.*
- *Ensures that services provided are consistent with the mission, purposes, and goals of the service.*
- *Ensures that services are provided in accordance with established policies and procedures.*
- *Reviews and updates policies and procedures.*
- *Provides training that assures continued competence of physical therapy support personnel.*
- *Provides for continuous in-service training on safety issues and for periodic safety inspection of equipment by qualified individuals.*

E. Fiscal Management
The director of the physical therapy service, in consultation with staff and appropriate administrative personnel, is responsible for planning for, and allocation of, resources. Fiscal planning and management of the service is based on sound accounting principles.

Criteria
The fiscal management plan includes:
- *Preparation and monitoring of a budget that provides for optimum use of resources.*
- *Accurate recording and reporting of financial information.*
- *Conformance with legal requirements.*
- *Cost-effective utilization of resources.*
- *A fee schedule that is consistent with cost of services and that is within customary norms of fairness and reasonableness.*

F. Quality/Performance Improvement
The physical therapy service has a written plan for continuous improvement of the performance of services provided.

Criteria:
The plan:
- *Provides evidence of ongoing review and evaluation of the service.*
- *Provides a mechanism for documentation of performance improvement.*

- *Is consistent with requirements of external agencies, if applicable.*

G. Staffing
The physical therapy personnel affiliated with the physical therapy service have demonstrated competence and are sufficient to achieve the mission, purposes, and goals of the service.

Criteria
The service:
- *Meets all legal requirements regarding licensure and/or certification of appropriate personnel.*
- *Provides staff expertise that is appropriate to the patients/clients served.*
- *Provides for appropriate staff-to-patient/client ratios.*
- *Provides for appropriate ratios of support staff to professional staff.*

H. Staff Development
The physical therapy service has a written plan that provides for appropriate and ongoing staff development.

Criteria
The plan:
- *Provides for consideration of self-assessments, individual goal setting, and organization needs in directing continuing education and learning activities.*
- *Includes strategies for long-term learning and professional development.*

I. Physical Setting
The physical setting is designed to provide a safe and accessible environment that facilitates fulfillment of the mission and achievement of the purposes and goals of the physical therapy service. The equipment is safe and sufficient to achieve the purposes and goals of physical therapy.

Criteria
The physical setting:
- *Meets all applicable legal requirements for health and safety.*
- *Meets space needs appropriate for the number and type of patients/clients served.*

The equipment:
- *Meets all applicable legal requirements for health and safety.*
- *Is inspected routinely.*

J. Interdisciplinary Collaboration
The physical therapy service collaborates with all appropriate disciplines.

Criteria
The collaboration includes:
- *An interdisciplinary team approach to patient/client care.*
- *Interdisciplinary patient/client and family education.*
- *Interdisciplinary staff development and continuing education.*

III. PROVISION OF SERVICES

A. Informed Consent

The physical therapist has sole responsibility for providing information to the patient/client and for obtaining the patient's/client's informed consent in accordance with jurisdictional law before initiating physical therapy.

Criteria

The information provided to the patient/client should include the following:
- *A clear description of the proposed intervention/treatment.*
- *A statement of material (decisional) risks associated with the proposed intervaention/ treatment.*
- *A statement of expected benefits of the proposed intervention/ treatment.*
- *A comparison of the benefits and risks possible both with and without intervention/ treatment.*
- *An explanation of reasonable alternatives to the recommended intervention/treatment.*

Informed consent requires:
- *Consent by a competent adult.*
- *Consent by a parent/legal guardian as the surrogate decision maker when the adult patient/client is not competent or when the patient/client is a minor.*

The patient's/client's acknowledgment of understanding and consent before the intervention/ treatment proceeds.

B. Initial Examination and Evaluation

The physical therapist performs and documents an initial examination and evaluates the results to identify problems and determine the diagnosis prior to intervention/treatment.

Criteria

The examination:
- *Is documented, dated, and signed by the physical therapist who performed the examination.*
- *Identifies the physical therapy needs of the patient/client.*
- *Incorporates appropriate objective tests and measures to facilitate outcome measurement.*
- *Documents sufficient data to establish a plan of care.*
- *May result in recommendations for additional services to meet the needs of the patient/client.*

C. Plan of Care

The physical therapist establishes and provides a plan of care for the individual based on the results of the examination and evaluation and on patient/client needs.

The physical therapist involves the patient/client and appropriate others in the planning, implementation, and assessment of the intervention/treatment program.

The physical therapist, in consultation with appropriate disciplines, plans for discharge of the patient/ client taking into consideration goal achievement, and provides for appropriate follow-up or referral.

Criteria

The plan of care includes:
- *Realistic goals and expected functional outcomes.*
- *Intervention/treatment, including its frequency and duration.*

- *Documentation that is dated and signed by the physical therapist who established the plan of care.*

D. Intervention/Treatment

The physical therapist provides, or delegates and supervises, the physical therapy intervention/ treatment consistent with the results of the examination and evaluation and plan of care.

The physical therapist documents, on an ongoing basis, services provided, responses to services, and changes in status relative to the plan of care.

Criteria

The intervention/treatment is:
- *Provided under the ongoing personal care or supervision of the physical therapist.*
- *Provided in such a way that delegated responsibilities are commensurate with the qualifications and legal limitations of the physical therapy personnel involved in the intervention/treatment.*
- *Altered in accordance with changes in individual response or status.*
- *Provided at a level that is consistent with current physical therapy practice.*
- *Interdisciplinary when necessary to meet the needs of the patient/client.*

Documentation of the services provided includes:
- *Date and signature of the physical therapist and/or of the physical therapist assistant when permissible by law.*

E. Reexamination and Reevaluation

The physical therapist reexamines and reevaluates the individual continually and modifies or discontinues the plan of care accordingly.

Criteria

The physical therapist:
- *Periodically documents, dates, and signs the patient/client reexamination and modifications of the plan of care.*

F. Discharge/Discontinuation of Treatment or Intervention

The physical therapist discharges the patient/client from physical therapy intervention/treatment when the goals or projected outcomes for the patient/client have been met.

Physical therapy intervention/ treatment shall be discontinued when the goals are achieved, the patient/ client declines to continue care, the patient/client is unable to continue, or the physical therapist determines that intervention/treatment is no longer warranted.

Criteria

Discharge documentation shall include:
- *The patient's/client's status at discharge and functional outcomes/goals achieved.*
- *Dating and signing of the discharge summary by the physical therapist.*
- *When a patient/client is discharged prior to goal achievement, the patient's/client's status and the rationale for discontinuation.*

IV. EDUCATION

The physical therapist is responsible for individual professional development. The physical therapist assistant is responsible for individual career development.

The physical therapist participates in the education of physical therapist students, physical therapist assistant students, and students in other health professions. The physical therapist assistant participates in the education of physical therapist assistant students and other student health professionals.

The physical therapist educates and provides consultation to consumers and the general public regarding the purposes and benefits of physical therapy.

The physical therapist educates and provides consultation to consumers and the general public regarding the roles of the physical therapist and the physical therapist assistant.

Criteria
The physical therapist educates and provides consultation to consumers and the general public regarding the roles of the physical therapist, the physical therapist assistant, and other support personnel.

V. RESEARCH

The physical therapist applies research findings to p
and encourages, participates in, and promotes activit
that establish the outcomes of physical therapist
patient/client management.

The physical therapist supports collaborative and int
ciplinary research.

VI. COMMUNITY RESPONSIBILITY

The physical therapist demonstrates community resp
bility by participating in community and community
agency activities, educating the public, formulating p
policy, or providing pro bono physical therapy servic

Criteria
The physical therapist demonstrates community res
bility by participating in community and communi
agency activities; educating the public, including pre
tion and health promotion activities; formulating p
policy; or providing pro bono physical therapy serv

Standards:
Adopted by the House of Delegates
June 1980
Amended June 1985, June 1991, June 1996

Criteria:
Adopted by the Board of Directors
March 1993
Amended November 1994, March 1995

Code of Ethics

PREAMBLE

This *Code of Ethics* sets forth ethical principles for the physical therapy profession. Members of this profession are responsible for maintaining and promoting ethical practice. This *Code of Ethics*, adopted by the American Physical Therapy Association, shall be binding on physical therapists who are members of the Association.

Principle 1
Physical therapists respect the rights and dignity of all individuals.

Principle 2
Physical therapists comply with the laws and regulations governing the practice of physical therapy.

Principle 3
Physical therapists accept responsibility for the exercise of sound judgment.

Principle 5
Physical therapists seek remuneration for their services th
deserved and reasonable.

Principle 6
Physical therapists provide accurate information to the consu
about the profession and about those services they provid

Principle 7
Physical therapists accept the responsibility to protect the pu
and the profession from unethical, incompetent, or illegal

Principle 8
Physical therapists participate in efforts to address the health
needs of the public.

Adopted by the House of Delegates
June 1981

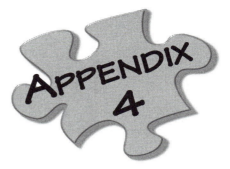

APPENDIX
4

GUIDE FOR PROFESSIONAL CONDUCT FOR THE APTA

The following is reprinted from APTA. *Guide for Professional Conduct of the Affiliate Member of the APTA*, with permission from the American Physical Therapy Association.

Guide for Professional Conduct

PURPOSE

This *Guide for Professional Conduct* (*Guide*) is intended to serve physical therapists who are members of the American Physical Therapy Association (Association) in interpreting the *Code of Ethics* (*Code*) and matters of professional conduct. The Guide provides guidelines by which physical therapists may determine the propriety of their conduct. The *Code* and the *Guide* apply to all physical therapists who are Association members. These guidelines are subject to changes as the dynamics of the profession change and as new patterns of health care delivery are developed and accepted by the professional community and the public. This *Guide* is subject to monitoring and timely revision by the Judicial Committee of the Association.

INTERPRETING ETHICAL PRINCIPLES

The interpretations expressed in this *Guide* are not to be considered all inclusive of situations that could evolve under a specific principle of the *Code* but reflect the opinions, decisions, and advice of the Judicial Committee. While the statements of ethical principles apply universally, specific circumstances determine their appropriate application. Input related to current interpretations, or to situations requiring interpretation, is encouraged from Association members.

PRINCIPLE 1

Physical therapists respect the rights and dignity of all individuals.

1.1 Attitudes of Physical Therapists

  A. Physical therapists shall recognize that each individual is different from all other individuals and shall respect and be responsive to those differences.
  B. Physical therapists are to be guided at all times by concern for the physical, psychological, and socioeconomic welfare of those individuals entrusted to their care.
  C. Physical therapists shall not engage in conduct that constitutes harassment or abuse of, or discrimination against, colleagues, associates, or others.

1.2 Confidential Information

  A. Information relating to the physical therapist/patient relationship is confidential and may not be communicated to a third party not involved in that patient's care without the prior written consent of the patient, subject to applicable law.
  B. Information derived from component-sponsored peer review shall be held confidential by the reviewer unless written permission to release the information is obtained from the physical therapist who was reviewed.
  C. Information derived from the working relationships of physical therapists shall be held confidential by all parties.
  D. Information may be disclosed to appropriate authorities when it is necessary to protect the welfare of an individual or the community. Such disclosure shall be in accordance with applicable law.

1.3 Patient Relations

  Physical therapists shall not engage in any sexual relationship or activity, whether consensual or nonconsensual, with any patient while a physical therapist/patient relationship exists.

1.4 Informed Consent

  Physical therapists shall obtain patient informed consent before treatment.

PRINCIPLE 2

Physical therapists comply with the laws and regulations governing the practice of physical therapy.

2.1 Professional Practice

  Physical therapists shall provide consultation, evaluation, treatment, and preventive care, in accordance with the laws and regulations of the jurisdiction(s) in which they practice.

PRINCIPLE 3

Physical therapists accept responsibility for the exercise of sound judgment.

3.1 Acceptance of Responsibility

  A. Upon accepting an individual for provision of physical therapy services, physical therapists shall assume the responsibility for evaluating that individual; planning, implementing, and supervising the therapeutic program; reevaluating and changing that program; and maintaining adequate records of the case, including progress reports.
  B. When the individual's needs are beyond the scope of the physical therapist's expertise, or when additional services are indicated, the individual shall be so informed and assisted in identifying a qualified provider.
  C. Regardless of practice setting, physical therapists shall maintain the ability to make independent judgments.
  D. The physical therapist shall not provide physical therapy services to a patient while under the influence of a substance that impairs his or her ability to do so safely.

3.2 Delegation of Responsibility

  A. Physical therapists shall not delegate to a less qualified person any activity which requires the unique skill, knowledge, and judgment of the physical therapist.
  B. The primary responsibility for physical therapy care rendered by supportive personnel rests with the supervising physical therapist. Adequate supervision requires, at a minimum, that a supervising physical therapist perform the following activities:
    1. Designate or establish channels of written and oral communication.
    2. Interpret available information concerning the individual under care.
    3. Provide initial evaluation.
    4. Develop plan of care, including short- and long-term goals.

C. Physical therapists should attempt to ensure that providers, agencies, or other employers adopt physical therapy fee schedules that are reasonable and that encourage access to necessary services.

5.2 Business Practices/Fee Arrangements

A. Physical therapists shall not:
1. directly or indirectly request, receive, or participate in the dividing, transferring, assigning, rebating of an unearned fee.
2. profit by means of a credit or other valuable consideration, such as an unearned commission, discount, or gratuity in connection with furnishing of physical therapy services.
B. Unless laws impose restrictions to the contrary, physical therapists who provide physical therapy services in a business entity may pool fees and moneys received. Physical therapists may divide or apportion these fees and moneys in accordance with the business agreement.
C. Physical therapists may enter into agreements with organizations to provide physical therapy services if such agreements do not violate the ethical principles of the Association.

5.3 Endorsement of Equipment or Services

A. Physical therapists shall not use influence upon individuals under their care or their families for utilization of equipment or services based upon the direct or indirect financial interest of the physical therapist in such equipment or services. Realizing that these individuals will normally rely on the physical therapists' advice, their best interest must always be maintained as well as their right of free choice relating to the use of any equipment or service. While it cannot be considered unethical for physical therapists to own or have a financial interest in equipment companies, or services, they must act in accordance with law and make full disclosure of their interest whenever such companies or services become the source of equipment or services for individuals under their care.
B. Physical therapists may be remunerated for endorsement or advertisement of equipment or services to the lay public, physical therapists, or other health professionals provided they disclose any financial interest in the production, sale, or distribution of said equipment or services.
C. In endorsing or adverting equipment or services, physical therapists shall use sound professional judgment and shall not give the appearance of Association endorsement.

5.4 Gifts and Other Considerations

A. Physical therapists shall not accept nor offer gifts or other considerations with obligatory conditions attached.
B. Physical therapists shall not accept or offer gifts or other considerations that affect or give an objective appearance of affecting their professional judgment.

PRINCIPLE 6

Physical therapists provide accurate information to the consumer about the profession and about those services they provide.

6.1 Information about the Profession

Physical therapists shall endeavor to educate the public to an awareness of the physical therapy profession through such means as publication of articles and participation in seminars, lectures, and civic programs.

6.2 Information about Services

A. Information given to the public shall emphasize that individual problems cannot be treated without individualized evaluation and plans/programs of care.
B. Physical therapists may advertise their services to the public.
C. Physical therapists shall not use, or participate in the use of, any form of communication containing a false, plagiarized, misleading, deceptive, unfair, or sensational statement or claim.
D. A paid advertisement shall be identified as such unless it is apparent from the context that it is a paid advertisement.

PRINCIPLE 7

Physical therapists accept the responsibility to protect the public and the profession from unethical, incompetent, or illegal acts.

7.1 Consumer Protection

A. Physical therapists shall report any conduct which appears to be unethical, incompetent, or illegal.
B. Physical therapists may not participate in any arrangements in which patients are exploited due to the referring sources enhancing their personal incomes as a result of referring for, prescribing, or recommending physical therapy.
C. Physical therapists shall be obligated to safeguard the public from underutilization or overutilization of physical therapy services.

7.2 Disclosure

The physical therapist shall disclose to the patient if the referring practitioner derives compensation from the provision of physical therapy. The physical therapist shall ensure that the individual has freedom of choice in selecting a provider of physical therapy.

PRINCIPLE 8

Physical therapists participate in efforts to address the health needs of the public.

8.1 Pro Bono Service

Physical therapists should render pro bono publico (reduced or no fee) services to patients lacking the ability to pay for services, as each physical therapist's practice permits.

Issued by Judicial Committee, APTA
October 1981
Last Amended September 1997

C. Physical therapists should attempt to ensure that providers, agencies, or other employers adopt physical therapy fee schedules that are reasonable and that encourage access to necessary services.

5.2 Business Practices/Fee Arrangements

A. Physical therapists shall not:
   1. directly or indirectly request, receive, or participate in the dividing, transferring, assigning, rebating of an unearned fee.
   2. profit by means of a credit or other valuable consideration, such as an unearned commission, discount, or gratuity in connection with furnishing of physical therapy services.
B. Unless laws impose restrictions to the contrary, physical therapists who provide physical therapy services in a business entity may pool fees and moneys received. Physical therapists may divide or apportion these fees and moneys in accordance with the business agreement.
C. Physical therapists may enter into agreements with organizations to provide physical therapy services if such agreements do not violate the ethical principles of the Association.

5.3 Endorsement of Equipment or Services

A. Physical therapists shall not use influence upon individuals under their care or their families for utilization of equipment or services based upon the direct or indirect financial interest of the physical therapist in such equipment or services. Realizing that these individuals will normally rely on the physical therapists' advice, their best interest must always be maintained as well as their right of free choice relating to the use of any equipment or service. While it cannot be considered unethical for physical therapists to own or have a financial interest in equipment companies, or services, they must act in accordance with law and make full disclosure of their interest whenever such companies or services become the source of equipment or services for individuals under their care.
B. Physical therapists may be remunerated for endorsement or advertisement of equipment or services to the lay public, physical therapists, or other health professionals provided they disclose any financial interest in the production, sale, or distribution of said equipment or services.
C. In endorsing or adverting equipment or services, physical therapists shall use sound professional judgment and shall not give the appearance of Association endorsement.

5.4 Gifts and Other Considerations

A. Physical therapists shall not accept nor offer gifts or other considerations with obligatory conditions attached.
B. Physical therapists shall not accept or offer gifts or other considerations that affect or give an objective appearance of affecting their professional judgment.

PRINCIPLE 6

Physical therapists provide accurate information to the consumer about the profession and about those services they provide.

6.1 Information about the Profession

Physical therapists shall endeavor to educate the public to an awareness of the physical therapy profession through such means as publication of articles and participation in seminars, lectures, and civic programs.

6.2 Information about Services

A. Information given to the public shall emphasize that individual problems cannot be treated without individualized evaluation and plans/programs of care.
B. Physical therapists may advertise their services to the public.
C. Physical therapists shall not use, or participate in the use of, any form of communication containing a false, plagiarized, fraudulent, misleading, deceptive, unfair, or sensational statement or claim.
D. A paid advertisement shall be identified as such unless it is apparent from the context that it is a paid advertisement.

PRINCIPLE 7

Physical therapists accept the responsibility to protect the public and the profession from unethical, incompetent, or illegal acts.

7.1 Consumer Protection

A. Physical therapists shall report any conduct which appears to be unethical, incompetent, or illegal.
B. Physical therapists may not participate in any arrangements in which patients are exploited due to the referring sources enhancing their personal incomes as a result of referring for, prescribing, or recommending physical therapy.
C. Physical therapists shall be obligated to safeguard the public from underutilization or overutilization of physical therapy services.

7.2 Disclosure

The physical therapist shall disclose to the patient if the referring practitioner derives compensation from the provision of physical therapy. The physical therapist shall ensure that the individual has freedom of choice in selecting a provider of physical therapy.

PRINCIPLE 8

Physical therapists participate in efforts to address the health needs of the public.

8.1 Pro Bono Service

Physical therapists should render pro bono publico (reduced or no fee) services to patients lacking the ability to pay for services, as each physical therapist's practice permits.

Issued by Judicial Committee, APTA
October 1981
Last Amended September 1997

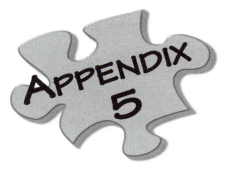

APPENDIX
5

GUIDE FOR CONDUCT OF THE AFFILIATE MEMBER OF THE APTA

The following is reprinted from APTA. *Guide for Conduct of the Affiliate Member of the APTA*, with permission from the American Physical Therapy Association.

Standards of Ethical Conduct for the Physical Therapist Assistant

PREAMBLE

Physical therapist assistants are responsible for maintaining and promoting high standards of conduct. These *Standards of Ethical Conduct for the Physical Therapist Assistant* shall be binding on physical therapist assistants who are affiliate members of the Association.

STANDARD 1

Physical therapist assistants provide services under the supervision of a physical therapist.

STANDARD 2

Physical therapist assistants respect the rights and dignity of all individuals.

STANDARD 3

Physical therapist assistants maintain and promote high standards in the provision of services, giving the welfare of the patients their highest regard.

STANDARD 4

Physical therapist assistants provide services within the limits of the law.

STANDARD 5

Physical therapist assistants make those judgments that are commensurate with their qualifications as physical therapist assistants.

STANDARD 6

Physical therapist assistants accept the responsibility to protect the public and the profession from unethical, incompetent, or illegal acts.

Adopted by House of Delegates
June 1982
Amended June 1991

Appendix 6

Guide for Conduct of the Affiliate Member

PURPOSE

This *Guide* is intended to serve physical therapist assistants who are affiliate members of the American Physical Therapy Association in the interpretation of the *Standards of Ethical Conduct for the Physical Therapist Assistant*, providing guidelines by which they may determine the propriety of their conduct. These guidelines are subject to change as new patterns of health care delivery are developed and accepted by the professional community and the public. This *Guide* is subject to monitoring and timely revision by the Judicial Committee of the Association.

INTERPRETING STANDARDS

The interpretations expressed in this *Guide* are not to be considered all inclusive of situations that could evolve under a specific standard of the *Standards of Ethical Conduct for the Physical Therapist Assistant* but reflect the opinions, decisions, and advice of the Judicial Committee. While the statements of ethical standards apply universally, specific circumstances determine their appropriate application. Input related to current interpretations, or to situations requiring interpretation, is encouraged from APTA members.

STANDARD 1

Physical therapist assistants provide services under the supervision of a physical therapist.

1.1 Supervisory Relationships

Physical therapist assistants shall work under the supervision and direction of a physical therapist who is properly credentialed in the jurisdiction in which the physical therapist assistant practices.

1.2 Performance of Service

A. Physical therapist assistants may not initiate or alter a treatment program without prior evaluation by and approval of the supervising physical therapist.

B. Physical therapist assistants may modify a specific treatment procedure in accordance with changes in patient status.

C. Physical therapist assistants may not interpret data beyond the scope of their physical therapist assistant education.

D. Physical therapist assistants may respond to inquiries regarding patient status to appropriate parties within the protocol established by a supervising physical therapist.

E. Physical therapist assistants shall refer inquiries regarding patient prognosis to a supervising physical therapist.

STANDARD 2

Physical therapist assistants respect the rights and dignity of all individuals.

2.1 Attitudes of Physical Therapist Assistants

A. Physical therapist assistants shall recognize that each individual is different from all other individuals and respect and be responsive to those differences.

B. Physical therapist assistants shall be guided at all times by concern for the dignity and welfare of those patients entrusted to their care.

C. Physical therapist assistants shall not engage in conduct that constitutes harassment or abuse of, or discrimination against, colleagues, associates, or others.

2.2 Request for Release of Information

Physical therapist assistants shall refer all requests for release of confidential information to the supervising physical therapist.

2.3 Protection of Privacy

Physical therapist assistants must treat as confidential all information relating to the personal conditions and affairs of the persons whom they serve.

2.4 Patient Relations

Physical therapist assistants shall not engage in any sexual relationship or activity, whether consensual or nonconsensual, with any patient while a physical therapist assistant/patient relationship exists.

STANDARD 3

Physical therapist assistants maintain and promote high standards in the provision of services, giving the welfare of patients their highest regard.

3.1 Information About Services

A. Physical therapist assistants may provide consumers with information regarding provision of services within the protocol established by a supervising physical therapist.
B. Physical therapist assistants may not use, or participate in the use of, any form of communication containing a false, fraudulent, misleading, deceptive, unfair, or sensational statement or claim.

3.2 Organizational Employment

Physical therapist assistants shall advise their employer(s) of any employer practice which causes them to be in conflict with the *Standards of Ethical Conduct for the Physical Therapist Assistant.*

3.3 Endorsement of Equipment

Physical therapist assistants may not endorse equipment or exercise influence on patients or families to purchase or lease equipment except as directed by a physical therapist acting in accord with the stipulation in paragraph 5.3.A. of the *Guide for Professional Conduct.*

3.4 Financial Considerations

Physical therapist assistants shall never place their own financial interest above the welfare of their patients.

3.5 Exploitation of Patients

Physical therapist assistants shall not participate in any arrangements in which patients are exploited. Such arrangements include situations where referring sources enhance their personal incomes as a result of referring for, delegating, prescribing, or recommending physical therapy services.

STANDARD 4

Physical therapist assistants provide services within the limits of the law.

4.1 Supervisory Relationships

Physical therapist assistants shall comply with all aspects of law. Regardless of the content of any law, physical therapist assistants shall provide services only under the supervision and direction of a physical therapist who is properly credentialed in the jurisdiction in which the physical therapist assistant practices.

4.2 Representation

Physical therapist assistants shall not hold themselves out as physical therapists.

STANDARD 5

Physical therapist assistants make those judgments that are commensurate with their qualifications as physical therapist assistants.

5.1 Patient Treatment

Physical therapist assistants shall report all untoward patient responses to a supervising physical therapist.

5.2 Patient Safety

A. Physical therapist assistants may refuse to carry out treatment procedures that they believe to be not in the best interest of the patient.
B. The physical therapist assistant shall not provide physical therapy services to a patient while under the influence of a substance that impairs his or her ability to do so safely.

5.3 Qualifications

Physical therapist assistants may not carry out any procedure that they are not qualified to provide.

5.4 Discontinuance of Treatment Program

Physical therapist assistants shall discontinue immediately any treatment procedures which in their judgment appear to be harmful to the patient.

5.5 Continued Education

Physical therapist assistants shall continue participation in various types of educational activities which enhance their skills and knowledge and provide new skills and knowledge.

STANDARD 6

Physical therapist assistants accept the responsibility to protect the public and the profession from unethical, incompetent, or illegal acts.

6.1 Consumer Protection

Physical therapist assistants shall report any conduct which appears to be unethical or illegal.

Issued by Judicial Committee, APTA
October 1981
Last Amended January 1996

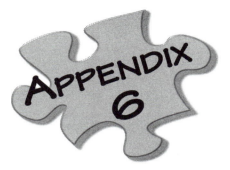

DIRECTION, DELEGATION, AND SUPERVISION IN PHYSICAL THERAPY SERVICES

The following is reprinted from APTA. *Direction, Delegation, and Supervision in Physical Therapy Services*, with permission from the American Physical Therapy Association.

American Physical Therapy Association

DIRECTION, DELEGATION, AND SUPERVISION IN PHYSICAL THERAPY SERVICES

HOD 06-96-30-42 (Program 32)
[Amended HOD 06-95-11-06; HOD 06-93-08-09; HOD 06-85-20-41;
Initial HOD 06-84-16-72/HOD 06-78-22-61/HOD 06-77-19-37]

Physical therapists have a responsibility to deliver services in ways that protect the public safety and maximize the availability of the services. They do this through direct delivery of services in conjunction with responsible delegation of certain tasks to physical therapist assistants, physical therapy aides, and other support personnel.

Direction and supervision are essential in the provision of high-quality physical therapy services. The degree of direction and supervision necessary for ensuring high-quality physical therapy services is dependent on many factors, including the education, experience, and responsibilities of the parties involved as well as the organizational structure in which the physical therapy services are provided. Supervision should be readily available to the individual being supervised.

The director of a physical therapy service is a physical therapist who has demonstrated qualifications based on education and experience in the field of physical therapy and who has accepted the inherent responsibilities. The director of a physical therapy service must: (1) establish guidelines and procedures that will delineate the functions and responsibilities of all levels of physical therapy personnel in the service and the supervisory relationships inherent to the functions of the service and the organization; (2) ensure that the objectives of the service are efficiently and effectively achieved within the framework of the stated purpose of the organization and in accordance with safe physical therapy practice; and (3) interpret administrative policies, act as a liaison between line staff and administration, and foster the professional growth of the staff.

Written standards of practice and performance criteria should be available for all levels of physical therapy personnel in a physical therapy service. Regularly scheduled performance appraisals should be conducted by the supervisor based on these standards of practice and performance criteria.

Delegated responsibilities must be commensurate with the qualifications, including experience, education, and training, of the individuals to whom the responsibilities are being assigned. When the physical therapist of record delegates patient care responsibilities to physical therapist assistants or other support personnel, that physical therapist holds responsibility for supervision of the physical therapy program. Regardless of the setting in which the service is given, the following responsibilities must be borne solely by the physical therapist:

1. Interpretation of referrals when available.
2. Initial evaluation, problem identification, and diagnosis for physical therapy.
3. Development or modification of a plan of care which is based on the initial evaluation and which includes the physical therapy treatment goals.
4. Determination of which tasks require the expertise and decision-making capacity of the physical therapist and must be personally rendered by the physical therapist, and which tasks may be delegated. Prior to delegating any procedure, the physical therapist should determine that the consequences of the procedure are predictable, the situation is stable, and the basic indicators are not ambiguous and do not require ongoing observation by the physical therapist.
5. Delegation and instruction of the services to be rendered by the physical therapist assistant or other support personnel, including, but not limited to, specific treatment program, precautions, special problems, and contraindicated procedures.
6. Timely review of treatment documentation, reevaluation of the patient and the patient's treatment goals, and revision of the plan of care when indicated.
7. Establishment of the discharge plan and documentation of discharge summary/status.

A. Definition and Utilization of the Physical Therapist Assistant

Definition
The physical therapist assistant is a technically educated health care provider who assists the physical therapist in the provision of physical therapy. The physical therapist assistant is a graduate of a physical therapist assistant associate degree program accredited by an agency recognized by the Secretary of the US Department of Education or the Council on Postsecondary Accreditation.

Utilization
The physical therapist of record is the person who is directly responsible for the actions of the physical therapist assistant. The physical therapist assistant may perform physical therapy procedures and related tasks that have been selected and delegated by the supervising physical therapist. Where permitted by law, the physical therapist assistant may also carry out routine operational functions, including supervision of the physical therapy aide and documentation of treatment progress. The ability of the physical therapist assistant to perform the selected and delegated tasks shall be assessed on an ongoing basis by the supervising physical therapist. The physical therapist assistant may modify a specific treatment procedure in accordance with changes in patient status within the scope of the established treatment plan.

The physical therapist assistant must work under the direction and supervision of the physical therapist in all practice settings. When the physical therapist and the physical therapist assistant are not within the same physical setting, the performance of the delegated functions by the physical therapist assistant must be consistent with safe and legal physical therapy practice and shall be predicated on the following factors: complexity and acuity of the patient's needs, proximity and accessibility to the physical therapist, supervision available in the event of emergencies or critical events, and type of setting in which the service is provided. When the physical therapist and the physical therapist assistant are not continuously within the same physical setting, greater emphasis in directing the physical therapist assistant must be placed on oral and written reporting.

When supervising the physical therapist assistant in any off-site setting, the following requirements must be observed:
1. A qualified physical therapist must be accessible by telecommunications to the physical therapist assistant at all times while the physical therapist assistant is treating patients.
2. The initial visit must be made by a qualified physical therapist for evaluation of the patient and establishment of a plan of care.
3. There must be regularly scheduled and documented conferences with the physical therapist assistant regarding patients, the frequency of which is determined by the needs of the patient and the needs of the physical therapist assistant.
4. In those situations in which a physical therapist assistant is involved in the care of a patient, a supervisory visit by the physical therapist will be made:
    a. On the physical therapist assistant's request for a reevaluation, when a change in treatment plan of care is needed, prior to any planned discharge, and in response to a change in the patient's medical status.
    b. At least once a month, or at a higher frequency when established by the physical therapist, in accordance with the needs of the patient.
    c. A supervisory visit should include:
        1. An on-site reassessment of the patient.
        2. On-site review of the plan of care with appropriate revision or termination.
        3. Assessment and recommendation for utilization of outside resources.

B.   Definition and Utilization of the Physical Therapy Aide

Definition

The physical therapy aide is a nonlicensed worker who is specifically trained under the direction of a physical therapist. The physical therapy aide performs designated routine tasks related to the operation of a physical therapy service delegated by the physical therapist or, in accordance with the law, by a physical therapist assistant.

Utilization

The physical therapist of record is the person who is directly responsible for the actions of the physical therapy aide. The physical therapy aide provides support services in the physical therapy service, which may include patient related or non-patient-related duties. When providing direct physical therapy services to patients, the physical therapy aide may function only with the continuous on-site supervision of the physical therapist or, where allowable by law and/or regulation, the physical therapist assistant. Continuous on-site supervision requires the presence of the physical therapist or physical therapist assistant in the immediate area, and the involvement of the physical therapist or physical therapist assistant in appropriate aspects of each treatment session in which a component of treatment is delegated to a physical therapy aide.

The physical therapy aide may assist patients in preparation for treatment and, as necessary, during treatment and at the conclusion of treatment, and may assemble and disassemble equipment and accessories, in accordance with the training of the physical therapy aide. The extent to which the physical therapy aide participates in operational activities, including maintenance and transportation and in patient-related activities, will be dependent on the discretion of the physical therapist and the applicable state and federal regulations.

Students who are enrolled in physical therapist professional education programs or physical therapist assistant education programs and who are employed in a physical therapy clinical setting where such employment is not a part of the formal educational curriculum will be classified as physical therapy aides. Where their employment is part of the formal educational curriculum this policy will not apply. The physical therapist student who is a graduate of an approved physical therapist assistant program is exempt from this restriction and may be classified as a physical therapist assistant.

C.   Other Support Personnel

When other personnel (eg, exercise physiologists, athletic trainers, massage therapists) work within the setting of a physical therapy service they should be employed under their appropriate title. Any involvement in patient care activities should be within the limits of their education, in accordance with applicable laws and regulations, and at the discretion of the physical therapist. However, if they function as an extension of the physical therapist's license, their title and all provided services must be in accordance with state and federal laws and regulations. In all situations when the physical therapist delegates activities to other support personnel, the physical therapist must recognize the legal responsibility and liability for such delegation.

American Physical Therapy Association
1111 North Fairfax Street, Alexandria, VA 22314-1488

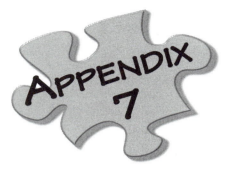

SAMPLE OF A CRITICAL (CLINICAL) PATHWAY

The following is reprinted with permission from St. Agnes Medical Center, Fresno, Calif; 1998.

SAINT AGNES MEDICAL CENTER, Fresno, CA →→*TOTAL KNEE CLINICAL PATHWAY*←← (Page 1, side 1)

CATEGORY	Pre-OP Date: / /	SURGERY DAY Date: / /	Post-Op Day 1 Date: / / 7A	Post-Op Day 2 Date: / / 7A
Cardiovascular Status (alteration in CV tissue perfusion)	VS q 8 hrs	VS q 4 hrs NeuroVascular check q 4 hrs	VS q 8 hrs NeuroVascular check q 4 hrs	VS q 8 hrs NeuroVascular check q 8 hrs
Respiratory (impaired gas exchange)		C&DB/IS q 1hr WA	C&DB/IS q 1hr WA	C&DB/IS q 8 hrs
Nutrition/ Elimination	Diet as tolerated Pt NPO at :	Diet as tolerated	Diet as tolerated	Diet as tolerated Monitor for BM
Activity				Up in chair /c leg extended - bid
NURSING (activity intolerance)	Up ad lib	Ensure CPM adjusted to fit Pt CPM: -5° hyperextension to 40° flexion	Up in chair /c leg extended - bid ↑CPM as tolerated	☆ **AMBULATE** ft /c [ ] walker or [ ] crutches: [ ] mod [ ] min [ ] CG assist ☆ **AMBULATE** ft /c [ ] walker or [ ] crutches: [ ] mod [ ] min [ ] walker or [ ] crutches: [ ] mod [ ] min [ ] CG assist ↑CPM as tolerated
Activity	*P.T. Brief History:*		**ACTIVITY GOALS:** ⇨ Ambulate: 0-10 feet ⇨ CPM Flexion: 90° by DC ⇨ PROM: -18 to 45° WB Status:	**ACTIVITY GOALS:** ⇨ Ambulate: 10-50 feet ⇨ CPM Flexion: 90° by DC ⇨ PROM: -15 to 60° WB Status:
PHYSICAL & OCCUPATIONAL THERAPY	*Definitions:* max - patient 25% mod - patient 50% min - patient 75% CGA (contact guard) - hold gait belt SBA (stand by) - available to assist	Previous pertinent surgery: [ ] THR [ ] right [ ] left [ ] TKR [ ] right [ ] left Other- Present ambulatory status: [ ] Walker [ ] Cane [ ] Crutches [ ] No Device Other - Walking tolerance: Other medical:	Teaching protocol done: AM___ PM___ **MORNING** ☆ [ ] STAND, [ ] AMB ft /c walker: [ ] max [ ] mod [ ] min assist Balance:___ Endurance:___ Bed Transfer/ Mobility /c [ ] max [ ] mod [ ] min assist PROM -5° to ___° ↑CPM -5° to ___° Subjective notes: **AFTERNOON** ☆ [ ] STAND, [ ] AMB ft /c walker: [ ] max [ ] mod [ ] min assist Balance:___ Endurance:___ Bed Transfer/ Mobility /c [ ] max [ ] mod [ ] min assist PROM -5° to ___° ↑CPM -5° to ___° Subjective notes:	Teaching protocol done: AM___ PM___ **MORNING** ☆ **AMBULATE** ft /c [ ] walker or [ ] crutches: [ ] mod [ ] min [ ] CG assist Balance:___ Endurance:___ Bed Transfer/ Mobility /c [ ] max [ ] mod [ ] min [ ] CG assist PROM ___° to ___° ↑CPM as tolerated -5° to ___ Subjective notes: **AFTERNOON** ☆ **AMBULATE** ft /c [ ] walker or [ ] crutches: [ ] mod [ ] min [ ] CG assist Balance:___ Endurance:___ Bed Transfer/ Mobility /c [ ] max [ ] mod [ ] min [ ] CG assist PROM ___° to ___° ↑CPM as tolerated -5° to ___ Subjective notes: Report to DP home equip needs & disch disposition [ ] Home Health [ ] SNF

Note: Individualization of patient care will occur based on each patient's clinical condition.   Rev. 3/15/96 (qrd) ver3

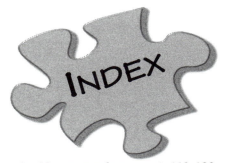